Weight-Loss Surgery Cookbook

SIMPLE AND DELICIOUS MEALS FOR
EVERY STAGE OF RECOVERY

CONTENTS

FOREWORD

Weight-loss surgery is a much-debated topic. Wherever you look in the media—in newspapers, on the Internet, on TV, on social networking sites like Facebook and Twitter—everyone seems to have something to say about it. And while it's fantastic that awareness is being raised and important issues are being discussed, this barrage of opinions can lead to misconceptions and confusion among the public and those who might be considering the surgery.

The truth is that weight-loss surgery has never been more popular or more successful at helping obese people lose significant amounts of weight on a permanent basis. It rightly deserves to be perceived as a hugely positive procedure, helping people to live longer, happier, and healthier lives.

The *Weight-Loss Surgery Cookbook* is all about demystifying the journey that bariatric surgery patients will travel after this life-changing operation. It lays out, in simple terms, the nutritional facts for those who are considering having a bariatric operation and provides useful information for those who have already undergone weight-loss surgery.

This book doesn't advise on which surgical procedure to choose—only your team of bariatric experts can do that. Instead, this is a nutrition and recipe book designed to help you maximize your success after surgery. It will rekindle enthusiasm in bariatrics who believe they might never eat normally again. It will show those who feel that they can't control their eating that, in fact, they can—with nutritious food, healthier choices, and support at every step of the way, regardless of their surgical procedure. It will help people learn that a new bariatric eating program will be low in fat and sugar, high in protein and fiber—as well as bursting with flavor and exciting new textures and tastes. The advice, tips, recipes, and cooking ideas on these pages will guide you through the post-surgery maze and make your experience as rich and rewarding as possible.

To put it simply, by following the information in this book, you will give yourself the very best chance of reaching your ultimate weight-loss goal.

INTRODUCTION

It's no secret that obesity is on the rise across the globe. It has now reached epidemic proportions; in fact, the prevalence of obesity nearly doubled between 1980 and 2008. According to figures from the World Health Organization (WHO) in 2008, more than 1.4 billion adults were overweight and half a billion were obese. Of these, a staggering 2.8 million people will die each year as a result of this obesity. It's not just a problem for adults, either; in 2008, more than 40 million preschool children around the world were overweight.

What Is Obesity?

Obesity is broadly defined as "abnormal or excessive fat accumulation that may impair health." The body mass index (BMI) is commonly used to classify whether an adult is overweight or obese—this is the weight in kilograms divided by the square of the height in meters. The WHO defines *overweight* as having a BMI of 25 or more, *obesity* as a BMI of 30 or more, and *morbid obesity* as a BMI of 40 or more.

What Causes Obesity?

The fundamental cause of obesity is an energy imbalance between calories consumed and calories burned. However, it's far more complicated than that.

Across the globe, people are eating more high-fat foods and engaging in less physical activity due to sedentary jobs and living in cities with numerous modes of transportation. Technological and sociological changes are contributing to the problem.

Genetics also play a part. In fact, genes are thought to be responsible for up to 70 percent of a person's weight gain, as they can control a person's appetite, satiety, and metabolism. Will power and lifestyle choices can also have a profound impact on a person's weight—so it's not a simple issue or a straightforward equation.

The Price of Obesity

The long list of severe health complications associated with obesity includes type 2 diabetes, high cholesterol, arthritis, high blood pressure, heart disease, depression, physical disabilities, and certain cancers.

At its simplest, obesity is highly disabling and can result in premature death. Factor in comorbidities, like diabetes and heart disease, and you can see that life can be shortened considerably through being overweight.

Physically, financially, and emotionally, the cost of obesity on an individual is very significant, but it's also costly to the nation. The economic costs through loss of work, additional health care needs, and incapacity benefits for those too ill to work are rising significantly.

Solutions

Anyone who has struggled with their weight will recognize that a lot of factors play a role in their weight management. It's naive to think that a "one size fits all" solution exists.

Research has shown us that diets often fail. Only a mere 5 percent of dieters lose their excess weight and keep it off long-term. The remaining 95 percent often yo-yo between one diet and the next, each time increasing their starting weight.

For some people, the final option is bariatric or weight-loss surgery. For those who have tried the usual, traditional methods of weight loss without success, surgery may be the only solution.

Bariatric surgery has been proven to be the most effective and longest-lasting treatment for morbid obesity and many related conditions. There is also mounting evidence to suggest that it may be among the most effective treatments for metabolic diseases and conditions, including obstructive sleep apnea, high cholesterol, nonalcoholic fatty liver disease, hypertension, and type 2 diabetes.

Surgery for the morbidly obese goes way beyond weight loss, for not only are the comorbidities above improved, but joint disease, asthma, and fertility can also be dramatically improved or resolved.

Bariatric surgery can typically lead to a 50 percent loss of excess weight over five years. For gastric bypass patients this can be higher, up to an average of 65 percent to 70 percent.

What Is Weight-Loss Surgery?

Weight loss, or bariatric, surgery can be a gastric band, gastric bypass, gastric sleeve, duodenal switch, or other revision surgery. It should be viewed as the *beginning* of the solution to obesity, rather than an end in itself. The surgery is simply a tool to help with weight loss.

Anyone who thinks the operation itself is a "magic wand" or the "easy way out" or "cheating" is sadly mistaken. This couldn't be further from the truth. Surgery is just the start; what you do afterward is the real key to success. Unfortunately, weight loss isn't easy, with or without surgery. (If it were, we would all be slim!)

Many find that the really hard work, both emotionally and physically, begins after their operation. Patients have to learn a new way of eating, break bad habits and destructive patterns that hamper success, develop new coping skills, and become more active for a sustainably healthy life.

That's why it's crucial that you seek out support from friends, family, your bariatric medical team, and other weight-loss surgery patients during this challenging time. It's also the time to arm yourself with as much valuable advice as possible—including this book—to ensure success, both during the weight–loss days and later during the maintenance phase.

The Many Benefits of Weight Loss

As with any kind of major surgery, undergoing a bariatric operation is not without risk. However, the majority of patients would agree that the health rewards gained far outweigh the possible complications.

Losing weight does so much more than just get you into a pair of "skinny jeans." It can boost your fertility, improve your sex life, and improve or reverse conditions such as chronic pain, type 2 diabetes, sleep apnea, high blood pressure, and high cholesterol. You'll also feel much more energetic and confident.

The transformations you'll experience, both inside and out, will be dramatic. Take pleasure in doing the simple things that you never would have done before—enjoying a walk with your dog, sitting on the beach in a bathing suit, playing with your children, taking a ride at a theme park, easily belting up the buckle in your airplane seat, and reducing or simply doing away with a whole repertoire of medications.

As you work through this book, consider participating in support groups and forums. It has been shown that patients who get involved and engage with the bariatric community have far better outcomes.

You can't underestimate the importance of the journey you're about to take. Congratulations on taking the first step toward a brighter, better you!

How to Use This Book

This cookbook and the recipes in it have been specifically designed and developed to help you at every stage after weight-loss surgery. There's advice for the first stage, "Clear Liquids"; additional advice and recipes for the second stage, "Full Liquids"; the same for the third and fourth stages, "Pureed Foods" and "Soft Foods"; and more for the fifth and final stage, "Eating Well for Life."

If the recipe has been color-coded as suitable for your eating stage, then it can be considered for your eating plan, although in some cases the **WLS (weight–loss surgery) portion** may need to be pureed, finely chopped, or broken down to a smoother acceptable texture before serving.

However, people's tolerances vary greatly, so while an ingredient may be recommended or a recipe suggested as being appropriate for a specific stage of your diet progression, only you will know what foods you can tolerate and when you can best tolerate them.

In addition, you'll find a nutritional analysis breakdown with every recipe. It includes calories and protein, carbohydrate, and fat levels. All analyses are based on the normal or average portion size. The WLS portion size is listed as well. Obviously, if you're a post-surgery patient, you'll be eating smaller portions than the analyzed amounts, so you'll be having fewer calories and less protein, carbohydrates, and fat.

The recipes in the book have been chosen, appraised, and evaluated from discussions with WLS patients who have had gastric bands, gastric sleeves, gastric bypasses, and duodenal switches (or other revision surgery) at countless dieticians' meetings, support groups, and on forums. They take into account that some patients sail through postsurgery with almost no digestion problems from the word "go," while others find each new stage a challenge due to food sensitivity. There should be something for everyone here.

If your experience of postsurgery eating is challenging, don't be afraid to be flexible with the recipes. For example, if you find it difficult to tolerate beef, then try substituting turkey or chicken instead. It will usually work just as well. This book is all about making the new way of eating work for you.

A final word of caution: As noted earlier, gastric bypass patients may well be susceptible to "dumping syndrome" (see page 11). This condition, which is characterized by bloating, nausea, and abdominal pain, among other symptoms, can be the result of eating too much sugar or fat in one hit. Sugar is often the main culprit. The best advice here is to be proactive and become a relentless label reader, since sugar is found in some products that you would never expect. Sometimes it can also happen if you have a sensitivity to artificial sweeteners. Most people who have experienced it say it's so awful, they'll do anything they can to avoid it happening again. Heed their warning and keep your sugar and fat intake low by eating right with every bite!

1

THE BASICS OF BARIATRIC NOURISHMENT

Eating Less, Eating Right

Losing and keeping the pounds off after weight-loss surgery depends not just on eating less, but on eating the right foods, with the right nutrition, in the optimum amounts. But finding the foods you can eat—and, moreover, *want* to eat—and making the transition from your "old life" to a healthy new one can be challenging. Even if you know a great deal about nutrition, putting this into practice is hard.

From the early post-op days when you're on fluids, purees, and soft foods into what is called "Eating Well for Life," it's important to practice "mindful eating"—making sure that you eat right with every bite.

Ironically, this can often be easier in the early "honeymoon" stage after surgery, when you might not have any real appetite or hunger for food, than in the later stages, although there can be the danger of not eating or drinking enough. During this time you can maximize your weight–loss results by eating right and exercising regularly.

Protein will be your greatest priority during this time of your body's recovery—and it's fair to say always will be. Most patients are told to aim for 70 g per day to facilitate good healing.

Carbohydrates come next, and although the recommended amounts vary by surgical procedure as well as medical issue (like diabetes), 130 g per day is often quoted in bariatric surgery scientific literature. The goal here is to eat mostly complex carbohydrates, found in plant-based foods, and few simple carbohydrates, which have little to no nutritional value. Eating 130 g per day may sound overwhelming and most likely won't happen in the first few months after surgery, but it's certainly something to aim for at least 6 to 9 months post-op. Gastric bypass patients will also have to watch their sugar intake to avoid "dumping syndrome" (see page 11).

Fats, often labeled the bad guys, also have a place in your diet, but the amount fluctuates enormously according to your surgical procedure. Your mantra here is to steer clear of saturated fats, keeping the level down to under 5 g fat per 100 g.

Add to that advice about eating "5 a day" (that is, a combined five portions of fruit and vegetables), consuming enough fiber, hydrating well (at least 2 quarts of water per day), and taking multivitamins and other supplements, and you have a regimen that can be more than a little daunting.

Don't worry—you can handle it. The recipes and advice in this book will act as a springboard for your new bariatric lifestyle.

Recipes, however, are one thing and general eating is another. It's strongly recommended that patients become avid, if not fanatical, readers of package labels. Understand and be aware that food manufacturers add sugar, salt, and fat to foods to make them taste better. Check out the best nutritional options—take a little extra time in the market to find them, speak to other bariatrics on websites and forums for advice, and pass along your good finds at support groups so everyone can benefit.

So remember, it's not just about eating less—although you'll undoubtedly have a smaller plateful than your non-bariatric-surgery counterparts—but about nourishing yourself with inspiring, healthful foods to ensure long-term success.

Dumping Syndrome

Dumping syndrome refers to several symptoms that may occur following the surgical removal of some or all of the stomach. The symptoms, which usually present themselves after you eat, range from nausea to diarrhea to fainting. As many as 80 percent of gastric bypass patients experience dumping syndrome, but less than 5 percent have serious problems with it. As a general rule, the more of your stomach has been removed, the more likely you are to experience dumping syndrome.

Dumping happens when food (especially sugar) moves too quickly through the stomach and is "dumped" into the small intestine. The body has a tough time handling this rapid influx of sugar and responds by adding a large amount of fluid to the small intestine. This fluid is the cause of dumping symptoms. Thankfully, this doesn't usually require medical treatment.

There are two kinds of dumping: early and late. Both occur after a meal, especially after eating foods high in fat, carbohydrates, or sugar (both table and natural, like that found in fruit).

Early dumping occurs within 30 minutes of eating a meal. In addition to being triggered by high-fat, high-carbohydrate, and high-sugar foods, early dumping can occur by eating foods that are too hot or too cold, or drinking liquids during your meal. Early dumping symptoms include bloating, vomiting, diarrhea, heart palpitations, nausea, sweating, dizziness, and rapid heart rate.

Late dumping is a form of hypoglycemia (low blood sugar). When you ingest too much sugar, your now-smaller stomach doesn't digest it properly, so your intestines absorb and deposit too much of it into your bloodstream. Your body then compensates by releasing more insulin, which makes your blood sugar drop. Symptoms of late dumping include anxiety, heart palpitations, fainting, fatigue, diarrhea, rapid heart rate, a strong feeling of hunger, sweating, weakness, dizziness, and confusion.

As long as you don't stray from your prescribed bariatric diet, you shouldn't experience dumping syndrome. For this reason, many patients view it as a "blessing in disguise" since it helps them keep their diet on track.

Interestingly, some patients' tolerance for foods that might trigger dumping syndrome can change over time. Some find that several years out of surgery they can tolerate small amounts of foods they couldn't eat in their earlier days.

Liquids for Life

The importance of keeping well hydrated after weight-loss surgery cannot be stressed enough. Dehydration in patients is a very common problem and can be very serious. You should be aiming to drink 2½ to 3½ quarts of liquid a day. Liquid is life's essential source for guaranteeing the body can run smoothly—so a drink should never be far from your side.

Water is the best possible choice, but to keep things varied, you can also go for well-diluted low-sugar juices or flavored waters with a very low sugar content. Sugar-free ice pops or ones made at home using low-sugar juice are also great, particularly in the summer.

Tea and coffee can be counted toward your daily liquid amount, but opt for decaffeinated herbal or fruit versions as caffeine is dehydrating in large quantities. Low-fat milk also counts as part of your liquid intake and is also a good source of protein.

Although deemed healthy, fruit juices can be very high in sugar, so be careful with these. Dilute them considerably—at least with the same quantity of water whenever possible. Salty drinks should also be kept to just 1 cup a day.

Protein drinks made from whey protein isolate, reconstituted with low-fat milk or water, are another option. Look for ones that are low in fat and sugar.

We also take in liquids via food. Fresh produce like vegetables and fruit, as well as fish and eggs, have a high water content and should be incorporated into your diet.

Signs of dehydration include:

- Dry, sticky mouth
- Darker than straw-colored urine
- Headache
- Decreased urination
- Thirst
- Dizziness or light-headedness

Not all liquids are good, either. Here are some to avoid:

- **Carbonated drinks and sodas:** These will make you bloated and are particularly bad for weight-loss surgery patients as they are capable of stretching your new stomach pouch. They can give you gas, chest pain, and uncomfortable pressure—so do yourself a favor and avoid them. If you really have no other option, be sure to add some ice cubes and swirl them around before drinking to get rid of as many bubbles as possible.
- **Alcohol:** Some surgeons say that alcohol is off-limits after weight-loss surgery; others say you can still drink, but in moderation and with caution. Since alcohol is absorbed straight from the stomach, and you now have a very small one, you'll find that alcohol affects you much faster than it used to. If you want to carry on drinking, just be cautious—drink very slowly and avoid carbonated beverages like mixers or beer. And don't forget that alcohol is full of empty calories and may prevent you from realizing your maximum weight-loss goal.

- **Energy drinks:** Many of these are promoted as healthy drinks or sports drinks, but this is very misleading as they are actually packed with sugar and caffeine. They can also cause dumping syndrome in gastric bypass patients (see page 11).
- **High-fat soups and drinks:** Rich and creamy soups, full-fat beverages like lattes and hot chocolate, and thick ice cream smoothies and milk shakes are high in calories and are best avoided. They can cause dumping in bypass patients (see page 11), particularly if the drinks are very hot or very cold. Duodenal switch patients may be at risk for loose stools due to impaired fat absorption, and band or sleeve patients can suffer because the fat content of these drinks delays stomach emptying.

The Five Stages of Eating After Bariatric Surgery

Surgical groups differ on some of their advice for eating after weight-loss surgery (and do follow your surgical team's advice to the letter, since they know you, the procedure you've had, and your medical background). They do, however, generally advocate five stages of eating:

- Stage 1: Clear Liquids
- Stage 2: Full Liquids
- Stage 3: Pureed Foods
- Stage 4: Soft Foods
- Stage 5: Eating Well for Life

Top Ten Tips from a Dietician

1. Keep to the five stages of postsurgery eating: Clear Liquids, Full Liquids, Pureed Foods, Soft Foods, and finally Eating Well for Life. Only progress to the next stage when you're completely comfortable with the current one and your surgeon has advised that it is safe to do so.

2. Chew, chew, and chew some more! Chewing your food well is key from the outset. Food should be cut into tiny pieces and chewed at least twenty times per mouthful. As time goes by, you'll be able to manage larger pieces of food, but chewing should stay thorough.

3. Relax, savor, and enjoy mealtimes with your friends and family.

4. Mealtimes shouldn't last more than half an hour, as grazing leads to over-consumption. It's a slippery slope if you get into the habit of eating until you're full, waiting for a bit, and then going back for more.

5. Eat three meals a day, plus two small, healthy snacks. Keep an eye on portion sizes by using a kitchen scale.

6. Keep your diet balanced and varied. Your main focus should be on making sure you eat enough protein, but carbohydrates and vegetables are important, too.

7. After gastric band surgery, patients should aim for 50 to 60 g of protein per day. After a bypass or gastric sleeve, patients should aim for 60 to 70 g per day; and after a duodenal switch, patients should aim for 80 to 120 g per day. Not meeting these levels could lead to hair loss and malnutrition.

8. Keep your fluids up. Drink enough liquid between meals to prevent dehydration. Aim for six to eight 8-fluid-ounce glasses every day. These should be noncaloric and decaffeinated. Do not drink immediately before, during, or after meals.

9. Take multivitamins and calcium supplements (plus any other supplements) as advised by your bariatric team or medical

practitioner. Follow these up with regular blood tests to check that your health is good.

10. Get cooking—it's the best way to know exactly what you're eating and control your diet while having an enriching, happy relationship with food.

Do You Know the 20:20:20 Rule?

You should aim to eat 20 mouthfuls of food for a meal, over a 20-minute period of time, chewing each mouthful 20 times, and putting your knife and fork down between each mouthful.

Try to eat mindfully at all times—eat your meals at the table or without distraction.

2

STAGE 1: CLEAR LIQUIDS

Eating Well in Stage 1

The first of the five post–bariatric surgery eating stages, and perhaps the most demanding, is known as Clear Liquids.

When you first return home from the hospital after your surgery, you'll be feeling tired, a little sore, and maybe a bit uncertain or daunted about what to eat or drink next. So it's important to be prepared in advance for this initial stage and follow your surgeon's advice and exact guidelines, which are personal to you. Depending on your situation, your doctor will recommend that you stick to clear fluids for just a few days or for as long as a month.

It's necessary to drink only fluids immediately after surgery in order to minimize digestion and your body's production of solid waste. This will ensure that your new gastrointestinal system is given the optimal chance to heal.

Clear liquids should be transparent, or "see-through," and thin enough to trickle through a sieve.

Guidelines recommend less than a 7-fluid-ounce portion at a time. **You should aim for 2½ to 3½ quarts of liquids per day—or at least 12 drinks.** This will seem like an awful lot to start with and hard to achieve, but keep at it. Spread your drinks out throughout the day and check your hydration by the color of your urine. If it's pale, you're drinking enough; if it's straw-colored or darker, this is a sign of dehydration, and you need to drink more.

You should have a drink by your side almost all the time in the early days to keep hydrated. Each beverage portion (1 portion = less than 7 fluid ounces) should be taken at least one hour apart, and sipped slowly, not gulped down in a rush. Slow and steady is the order of the day.

Listed below are some good examples of drinks from which to choose. Variety is crucial, so go for a mixture of sweet and savory drinks to avoid things getting boring. It's wise to start off with beverages that are at room temperature or warm before moving on to those that are hot, chilled, or iced.

Some of these drinks might taste strange to begin with, so dilute them with water or add ice to alter the concentration if it is too strong. Make some of your fluids nutritional so you stay well nourished. **Fizzy drinks are a real no-no and must be avoided at all times.**

Don't be tempted to move on to the next stage until you're advised to do so; otherwise you won't be ready.

Good Choices of Clear Liquids

- Plain, still water (not carbonated) or sugar-free flavored water
- Tea—warm traditional, fruit, spiced, herbal tea; or sugar-free iced tea
- Coffee—warm, ideally decaffeinated; or sugar-free iced coffee
- "No-added-sugar" or "sugar-free" juices
- "Salty" drinks diluted well with hot water
- Sugar-free ice pops
- Sugar-free Jell-O, made as per package instructions

- Chicken, beef, or vegetable stock, bouillon, broth, consommé, or clear soup
- Whey protein isolate fruit drink or low-fat and low-sugar protein drink supplement, made with water or milk—great for getting protein in the early days
- Low-fat milk or milk alternatives (see "Getting the Skinny on Milk Alternatives," below)

In addition, take a daily multivitamin and calcium supplement and any other supplements prescribed or recommended by your bariatric team.

Getting the Skinny on Milk Alternatives

Many pre-op, and most post-op, bariatric eating programs encourage drinking low-fat milk for its nutritional benefits of protein, high vitamins, and valuable mineral content. However, you may find this a tall order if you have lactose intolerance or insufficient lactase (the enzyme required to digest lactose, the natural sugar found in regular milk and dairy products) and suffer with bloating, gas, and changes in bowel habits.

Luckily, there are a variety of delicious and nutrient-packed milk alternatives available for those with such intolerances or allergies. Take a look at the healthy and tasty options below, but remember to choose and purchase the unsweetened variety to avoid excess sugar intake.

Soy milk: This is made by soaking dry soybeans and grinding them with water and sometimes some sugar. It's a good source of protein (about 7 g per 7 fluid ounces) and heart-healthy omega-3 fatty acids. It's often also fortified with calcium and vitamin D so it compares favorably with cow's milk. You could opt for a light soy milk (with less fat and lower calorie count), but remember it will have less protein in it, too.

Almond milk: This is made from ground almonds and filtered water and, like soy milk, is fortified with calcium and vitamin D. It's a thin milk with a nutty taste and great rich vitamin E content. The regular variety contains less protein than other milk alternatives (only about 1 g per 7 fluid ounces), but there is a protein-fortified version available that has 5 g per 7 fluid ounces, which may make it a better choice if protein is your priority.

Rice milk: This is a mixture of partially milled rice and water. Again, like almond milk, it has a thinner texture than ordinary milk, but also has a sweeter flavor. Lower in protein, too, at less than 1 g per 7 fluid ounces, it's a good choice for adding to breakfast cereals and in dessert recipes, providing you're meeting your protein needs with other foods.

Oat milk: Made from oats and water, this milk has a sweet, earthy flavor. It's a good source of protein (about 4 g per 7 fluid ounces) and is available fortified with calcium, vitamin A, and vitamin D. Oat milk generally has a higher sugar profile than other milk alternatives due to its natural starch content.

Hemp milk: This alternative is made from hemp seeds that have been soaked, then ground with water to make a creamy milk with a nutty taste. It has a moderate amount of protein (about 2 g per 7 fluid ounces), but is a great source of essential fatty acids and powerful antioxidants.

Coconut milk: This is milk made from the grated meat of the coconut and is usually fortified with vitamins A and D. It only has 1 g of protein per 7 fluid ounces (unless enriched with more) and does have a higher saturated fat level than other milk alternatives. It offers a good creamy texture but a distinctive tropical flavor, which works well with some recipes.

Staying the Course

This stage can be frustrating, but follow your bariatric team's advice and the guidelines in this chapter, and you'll be fine.

When your doctor gives you the green light, you'll be on to the next stage: Full Liquids.

3

STAGE 2: FULL LIQUIDS

Eating Well in Stage 2

Once you have completed the advised number of days drinking only clear liquids, you'll move on to stage 2, known as Full Liquids. This will probably come as a welcome relief and will offer you much more variety and a wider choice of flavors.

Full liquids are smooth and pourable. **They should be alternated with clear fluids throughout the day to ensure you stay hydrated.**

As with stage 1, your surgeon will tell you how many days of full liquids you should complete before moving on. Stage 2 is essential for preparing your new stomach for proper food, so getting into good habits now is really worth it in the long run.

You'll find this stage easier if you give yourself plenty of variation. Below is a list of good full liquids to choose from.

Good Choices of Full Liquids

- Milk—low-fat cow's, unsweetened soy, almond, rice, oat, hemp, or coconut (see "Getting the Skinny on Milk Alternatives," page 19)
- Milky chai-type tea, lightly spiced for added flavor

- Unsweetened plain (non-Greek-style) yogurt or yogurt without added sugar and fruit bits
- Low-fat and low-sugar whey protein isolate drinks—warm, cold, or icy, made with water or milk
- Whey protein isolate powder mixed with water or milk and made into an ice cream (see the Protein Ice Cream recipe on page 39)
- Mashed potato mixed with a little broth or gravy until thin and soup-like
- Diluted fruit juice
- Tomato or V8 juice—warm or chilled
- Homemade smoothies (but not too thick) or low-fat and low-sugar commercially made ones, diluted with water, if necessary
- Homemade cocoa (made with 2 teaspoons unsweetened cocoa powder and 7 fluid ounces low-fat milk) or low-fat and low-sugar hot chocolate
- Smooth cream-style (but not high-fat) soups
- Smooth cup-o-soups
- Homemade vegetable, fish, or poultry soups, pureed until smooth and diluted to a smooth, runny consistency
- Low-fat and low-sugar puddings
- Egg custards (very gently set)

Stocking Your New Pantry

It's so worthwhile to be well organized and have a fully stocked kitchen cupboard when you're following a bariatric eating program, as the food here will supplement the all-important fresh produce in your weekly grocery shopping. Depending on how much you liked to cook before your surgery, you may already have a lot of the ingredients listed below. On the other hand, some of these suggested staple foods might seem very new.

The foods listed below will allow you to make nutritious, healthy meals on short notice when there's no time to hit the store—making sure that you don't slip back into former bad habits. You'll also find that having some of the more unusual or luxurious ingredients on hand will allow you to make meals packed with flavor for more special occasions and when you're entertaining others. Stocking up your spice rack with a diverse selection of herbs and seasonings will also help with this.

Note that some weight–loss surgery patients will find they are intolerant of certain foods, such as artificial sweeteners, which can cause dumping syndrome (see page 11). Therefore, it's best to try new ingredients in small amounts before moving on to bigger portions.

Cans

- Beans (kidney, black, cannellini, flageolet, butter, low-sugar baked)
- Capers
- Chickpeas
- Coconut milk (reduced-fat)
- Consommé or broth (low-fat)
- Evaporated milk (light)
- Olives (green and ripe)
- Pudding (low-fat and low-sugar)
- Salmon (in oil or brine)
- Sardines (in brine or light tomato sauce)
- Tomatoes (chopped in juice)
- Tuna (in oil or brine)

Bottles, jars, and tubes

- Cooking sprays (low-fat)
- French dressing (fat-free or low-fat)
- Harissa paste
- Honey (clear)
- Horseradish and mint sauce
- Lime and lemon juice
- Low-sugar juices
- Mayonnaise (fat-free)

- Mustard (Dijon, English, and whole-grain)
- Oils (all types)
- Pesto sauce
- Pickled vegetables (low-sugar, like onions, gherkins, and dills)
- Soy sauce
- Tahini
- Tapenade
- Thai red and green curry paste
- Tomato ketchup (low-sugar)
- Tomato puree (double-concentrated)
- Tomato sauce and salsa (low-sugar)
- Vanilla extract or vanilla pods
- Vinegars (all types)
- Worcestershire sauce

Packages and cartons

- Amaretti cookies
- Bran cereal
- Bouillon cubes
- Cocoa powder (unsweetened)
- Cornstarch
- Deli or tortilla wraps (low-carb, traditional, or multigrain)
- Dried apricots
- Hot chocolate mix (low-fat and low-sugar)
- Jell-O (sugar-free)
- Lentils (green, red, and Puy)
- Low-fat milk powder
- Melba toast
- Muesli (low-sugar)
- Multigrain crispbreads and bread sticks
- Passata (crushed tomatoes)
- Porridge oats
- Rice (basmati, wild, and brown)
- Splenda granulated sweetener or other granulated sweetener of choice
- Unsalted nuts and trail mix
- Whole-wheat pita breads
- Whole-wheat pasta (spaghetti and shapes)

Chilled and dairy foods

- Babybel light cheese
- Butter (regular and light)
- Cheddar cheese (low-fat or reduced-fat)
- Cottage cheese (low-fat)
- Cream cheese or soft cheese (low-fat)
- Crème fraîche (reduced-fat)
- Eggs
- Egg whites
- Feta cheese
- Greek yogurt (fat-free)
- Halloumi cheese
- Hummus (reduced-fat)
- Laughing Cow light cheese wedges
- Milk (low-fat) or milk alternative
- Mozzarella (low-fat or half-fat)
- Parmesan cheese
- Ricotta (low-fat or half-fat)
- Spreads (low-fat)
- Whipped cream (low-fat)
- Yogurt (low-fat and low-sugar)

Chilled or frozen foods

- Bacon (traditional and turkey bacon)
- Beef, pork, and lamb filets or tenderloin
- Chicken and turkey thighs and breasts (skinless)
- Dressed crab
- Fish steaks and fillets
- Frozen peas, sweet corn, and stir-fry mixes
- Frozen raspberries and summer fruit mix
- Ground beef, lamb, and pork (extra-lean)
- Ground chicken and turkey
- Scallops
- Shrimp
- Smoked fish fillets
- Thin deli-sliced lean meats like ham, chicken, and turkey
- Tofu
- Veggie burgers or other meat alternatives (such as Quorn)

Special products

- Crystal Light lemonade crystals
- Protein whey isolate powders (flavored and unflavored, low-fat and low-sugar)
- Ready-made protein drinks (low-fat and low-sugar)

Dear Food Diary: Your Bariatric Journal

Keeping a food diary can be one of the most effective tools to track your food input (and to keep an accurate tally), and can also help to stop you from emotional eating. The power of the pen is mightier than the fork!

For bariatrics, this shouldn't just mean recording the types and amounts of food you're eating on a daily basis. It also means recording the feelings you experienced when eating that food. A bariatric journal is all about identifying the reasons some of us feel the need to eat when we aren't hungry and why. This will help you to make connections between your emotions and the foods that you have been using to satisfy them.

For example, you might have gotten into the habit of reaching for a chocolate bar whenever you have a fight with your partner or polishing off a package of cookies to take your mind off a stressful meeting coming up at work. These sorts of treats make us feel better while we are eating them—and we wrongly perceive them as giving us a bit of a "lift."

Understanding the connection between these unhealthy foods can help you create a strategy for stopping these urges. Begin by training yourself to reach for a healthy snack, such as an apple with some no-added-sugar peanut butter, instead of junk food the next time your emotions get the better of you.

A bariatric journal works as a visual aid and monitoring tool to show just how much, when, and where you are eating. It should include the date, time, food or beverage you're consuming, and what portion size.

The most important thing is to be honest with yourself—don't write down that you had a third of a tub of hummus when you had closer to half. You will only be cheating yourself in the long run. It's much better to tell the truth, and even if you have a splurge or binge, just write it down and aim for better tomorrow. No one is judging you.

Your journal could be a traditional notebook or you might like to consider one of the electronic food tracking websites or mobile phone apps out there, such as myfitnesspal.com. These are very convenient and really ingenious for working out the number of calories and grams of sugar or fat you have consumed at the click of a button—and they don't take up any extra space in your purse. Independent of or coupled with an exercise journal, they can monitor your weight-loss surgery journey more accurately, and on a day-to-day basis, than many other diagnostic tools. They also have a great memory so that you can look back and check just how far you have come.

Breakfasts: Getting a Great Early Start

A nutritious breakfast every day is a must for any bariatric patient. It's essential for kick-starting your metabolism and setting you up for the day ahead.

All of the choices below are protein-rich, quick, and easy to prepare, and some are suitable for eating on the move, too.

Breakfast Ideas for Stage 2

- Thin porridge made with low-fat milk
- Instant cereal made with low-fat milk
- Fruit smoothie diluted with water to a thin consistency
- No-added-sugar fruit juice diluted with water
- Low-fat and low-sugar whey protein isolate shake or protein drink
- Milky chai tea or low-fat and low-sugar chocolate drink
- Vanilla egg custards

Lunches: Some Light Bites

Lunch can often be the most difficult meal of the day to get right for bariatrics, as so many of us work in an office or are out and about at lunchtime. Here are some light-bite lunches to choose from—whether at home or at work. A thermos or microwave is all you need for the hot options, and a keep-cool lunchbox will work for the chilled ones.

Lunch Ideas for Stage 2

- Small cup of clear or pureed soup
- Low-fat and low-sugar smoothie
- Pureed or well-mashed smooth avocado with seasoning
- Mashed or pureed smooth tofu with vegetarian gravy

- Tender cooked lentils or dal thinned to a runny consistency
- Smooth cup-o-soup
- Very gently set egg custard
- Low-fat and low-sugar whey protein isolate drink or shake
- Low-fat and low-sugar sorbet or ice cream
- Low-fat and low-sugar mousse or yogurt
- Low-fat and low-sugar pudding with a little smooth pureed fruit

Full Liquids Stage Recipes

- Coffee Pumpkin Latte (page 31)
- Soy Chai Soother (page 32)
- Fruity Sipper (page 33)
- Cottage Mango Lassi (page 34)
- Back to Your Roots Juice (page 35)
- Tomato and Lentil Soup (page 36)
- Carrot, Lentil, and Bacon Soup (page 37)
- Forest Fruit and Apple Ice Pops (page 38)
- Protein Ice Cream (page 39)
- Vanilla Egg Custard (page 40)

Coffee Pumpkin Latte

Vegetarian

This is just the kind of warming cupful to enjoy when the colder autumn mornings begin or when you yearn for something warm and soothing in the early days after surgery. Use canned pure pumpkin for this recipe, not sweetened and seasoned pumpkin pie filling.

- 1 cup hot coffee
- 2 tablespoons canned pure pumpkin

- 1 cup unsweetened almond milk, warmed
- ¼ teaspoon pumpkin pie spice
- Sweetener, such as Splenda

In a warmed jug, whisk together ⅓ cup of the coffee with the pumpkin, almond milk, pumpkin pie spice, and sweetener to taste. Alternatively, mix in a blender.

Carefully pour the remaining coffee into a tall, heatproof glass, then add the pumpkin-coffee mixture so that it swirls throughout the glass.

Serve at once.

Serves 1

WLS portion ½ to 1

Calories per portion 53

Protein 2 g

Carbohydrate 6 g

Fat 2.7 g

Soy Chai Soother

Vegetarian

Here is a wonderfully soothing and lightly spiced chai tea, perfect for even the earliest of postsurgery days. You can choose any flavor of teabag (or loose tea, if you prefer to use a strainer), but Darjeeling is especially good.

- ⅔ cup water
- 1 teabag
- ½ teaspoon honey
- 2 to 3 drops vanilla extract
- 1 (3-inch) cinnamon stick, or ½ teaspoon ground cinnamon
- ½ teaspoon ground cardamom
- ¼ teaspoon ground ginger
- 1 whole clove
- ⅓ cup fat-free unsweetened soy milk

Place the water, teabag, honey, vanilla, cinnamon, cardamom, ginger, and clove in a small saucepan. Bring to the boil, then reduce the heat to maintain a simmer and simmer for about 3 minutes.

Remove from the heat and add the soy milk. Cover and leave to stand for 2 minutes to allow the spices to flavor the tea.

Strain the tea through a fine-mesh strainer into a bowl to remove the teabag, cinnamon stick, and any large particles of spices; discard the solids in the strainer. Transfer the chai to a mug and serve while still warm.

Serves 1

WLS portion ½ to 1

Calories per portion 54

Protein 2.7 g

Carbohydrate 5.8 g

Fat 1.6 g

Fruity Sipper

Vegan / Vegetarian / Suitable for Freezing

A well-diluted smoothie makes a good meal-in-a-glass option to sip during the early stages of eating after surgery. This one is bursting with flavor, vitamins, and antioxidants. It would also make a great liquid breakfast for those farther down the road of recovery.

- 1 medium banana
- 1½ cups strawberries, hulled (see tip, below)
- ¾ cup blueberries

- 2½ cups no-added-sugar pomegranate juice or red grape juice
- Crushed ice (optional)

Cut the banana into chunks and place in a blender with the strawberries, blueberries, and pomegranate or red grape juice. Blend on high power until smooth.

Add crushed ice, if desired, to make a seriously chilled drink. Transfer to a glass and serve at once.

Serves 4

WLS portion ½ to 1

Calories per portion 123

Protein 1.1 g

Carbohydrate 29.3 g

Fat 0.2 g

TIP

To save on preparation time, try freezing equal quantities of peeled, chopped bananas, blueberries, and hulled strawberries (or other fruits) in zip-top bags in the freezer for early-morning smoothie making. Blend while still frozen with juice or milk for a superchilled drink. You can also use store-bought frozen fruit with no added sugar or preservatives.

Cottage Mango Lassi

Vegetarian

There is no doubt that it is better to get your protein from food rather than supplements, which is why many dieticians steer clear of protein shakes. Adding cottage cheese to a drink (rather than protein powder) is a good solution to the need for an additional protein boost. Blend on high power to ensure the cottage cheese is processed to a smooth consistency.

- 1 cup fat-free unsweetened vanilla soy milk (or other low-fat milk)
- 2 tablespoons sugar-free vanilla syrup, or 1 to
- 2 teaspoons sweetener (such as Splenda)
- ¼ cup low-fat cottage cheese
- ¼ cup frozen mango chunks

Place the milk, syrup, cottage cheese, and mango chunks in a food processor or blender. Blend on high power until smooth.

Pour into a chilled glass and serve at once.

Serves 1

WLS portion: ½ to 1

Calories per portion 235

Protein 16.4 g

Carbohydrate 39.3 g

Fat 1 g

TIP

Fat-free Greek yogurt, frozen into cubes, can be used instead of cottage cheese, if preferred. Fresh mango cubes can also be used instead of frozen, but if using fresh mango, add a few ice cubes to the blender so that the mixture thickens to a smoothie or milk shake consistency.

Back to Your Roots Juice

Vegan / Vegetarian

In the early days after weight-loss surgery, it's imperative to get lots of fluids, but there is only so much water a person can endure. Alternating flavored water with teas, broths, smoothies, and shakes makes this more doable, but also consider some homemade juices made from fruits and vegetables. This beet, carrot, and radish option has the sweet addition of apples to make it drinkable at any time of day.

- 1 raw beet, scrubbed, trimmed, and chopped
- 2 carrots, chopped
- 10 French breakfast radishes, trimmed
- 2 apples, cored and chopped
- Flesh of ½ lemon, seeds removed

Place all the ingredients in a juicer and process to make a smooth juice.

Chill before serving.

Serves 2

WLS portion ½ to 1

Calories per portion 88

Protein 2.9 g

Carbohydrate 28.8 g

Fat 0.6 g

Tomato and Lentil Soup

Vegan / Vegetarian / Suitable for Freezing

Don't be tempted to omit the fresh mint from this recipe; it gives the soup a fresh, aromatic flavor to bring a change from what might become a repetitive bland soup scenario during the Full Liquids stage of eating. Puree the soup well and strain it in the very early stages after surgery, if desired; in later stages, it can be left chunky for serving.

- Low-fat nonstick cooking spray
- 1 onion, chopped
- 1 garlic clove, crushed
- 1 (14-ounce) can chopped tomatoes
- 1 (14-ounce) can lentils
- Handful of fresh mint leaves, chopped
- 2½ cups vegetable stock
- Salt and freshly ground black pepper

Spritz a large sauté pan with cooking spray. Add the onion and garlic and cook until softened, 3 to 5 minutes.

Add the chopped tomatoes and their juices, the lentils and their canning liquid, the mint, stock, and salt and pepper to taste. Bring to a boil, reduce the heat to maintain a simmer, cover, and simmer for 15 to 20 minutes.

Puree in a blender to serve smooth or serve chunky, if preferred, in the later stages of eating.

Serves 4

WLS portion ¼ to ½

Calories per portion 106

Protein 7.8 g

Carbohydrate 16.4 g

Fat 1.1 g

Carrot, Lentil, and Bacon Soup

Suitable for Freezing

This comforting soup is so easy to make and knocks the socks off any store-bought or ready-made variety. Not only is it easy on the wallet, but it can be frozen for up to three months. If you're pre-op, why not stash some away in small containers for when you come home after surgery? This is also a soup that is popular with the whole family, so it's worth making a large batch.

- Low-fat nonstick cooking spray
- 2 smoked bacon slices, chopped
- 1 large onion, chopped
- 1 pound carrots, chopped
- ½ cup raw red lentils
- 6 cups vegetable stock
- 1 tablespoon tomato paste
- 1 teaspoon medium-strength curry paste
- Salt and freshly ground black pepper
- 6 tablespoons fat-free Greek yogurt

Spritz a large sauté pan generously with cooking spray. Heat the pan over medium heat, add the bacon and onion, and cook for 4 to 5 minutes, or until the onion is pale golden.

Stir in the carrots, lentils, stock, tomato paste, curry paste, and salt and pepper to taste. Bring to a boil over medium-high heat and cook, uncovered, for 5 minutes. Reduce the heat to maintain a simmer, cover, and simmer for 20 minutes more, or until the carrots and lentils are tender.

Puree in a blender until smooth (be careful when blending hot liquids). Taste and adjust the seasoning, if necessary, then serve hot with a tablespoon of the yogurt swirled into each bowl of soup. (If you are making the soup ahead of time to freeze, omit the yogurt until serving.)

Serves 6

WLS portion ½ to ¾

Calories per portion 135

Protein 9.8 g

Carbohydrate 19.8 g

Fat 2 g

Forest Fruit and Apple Ice Pops

Vegan / Vegetarian / Suitable for Freezing

Somehow, in the very early stages after surgery, it seems easier to hydrate with an ice pop rather than a glass of fluid. Many commercial varieties, however, are too high in sugar and poor in nutrients. The answer is to make your own. Here is a fruit-laden option that is sure to please.

- 2 Pink Lady apples
- ¼ cup water
- 1 pound (or about a generous 3 cups) fresh or frozen mixed forest or summer berry

fruits (such as strawberries, blackberries, raspberries, and blackcurrants)
- 6 tablespoons Splenda granulated sweetener, plus more as needed

Peel, core, and chop the apples and place them in a large saucepan with the water. Set over moderate heat and cook for 4 minutes.

Add the berries and cook for 3 minutes more.

Remove from the heat and stir in the sweetener until dissolved. Taste and add a little more sweetener, if desired.

Puree in a blender, then strain through a fine-mesh sieve into a bowl to remove the seeds. Discard the solids in the sieve. Allow the puree to cool before pouring into ice-pop molds. Freeze overnight or for at least 6 hours until firm. Unmold to serve.

Serves 8

WLS portion 1

Calories per portion 33

Protein 0.7 g

Carbohydrate 7.3 g

Fat 0.1 g

Protein Ice Cream

Vegetarian / Suitable for Freezing

Many bariatric post-ops turn up their noses at flavored whey protein drink powders . . . but miraculously don't when they're made into an ice cream. Maybe this is because the drinks seem too sweet when made with milk or water at room temperature or chilled, but taste amazing frozen, when the sweetness diminishes. There's no doubt that an ice cream maker makes light work of this recipe, but it isn't essential. The hardest part is choosing a flavor—with so many varieties from chocolate chip to zesty lime, prepare yourself to be hooked on tasting a whole range of delicious ice creams. Nutritional guidelines have been calculated using a typical or average low-fat and low-sugar whey protein isolate flavored protein powder.

- 2¼ cups low-fat milk
- 4 (1-ounce) scoops flavored low-fat and low-sugar whey protein isolate powder in your flavor of choice

---

Mix the milk with the protein powder in a large jug, beating well to mix.

Pour the liquid into an ice cream maker and process according to the manufacturer's instructions until softly whipped and frozen. Spoon into one large or four small freezer containers and freeze until firm. You could serve softly frozen at this stage.

Alternatively, pour protein powder mixture into a large freezer container and freeze until firm, whisking once or twice during the process to break down any large ice crystals.

Remove from the freezer about 30 to 60 minutes before serving to soften slightly for scooping.

Serves 4

WLS portion ½ to 1

Calories per portion 133

Protein 27.2 g

Carbohydrate 6.3 g

Fat 0.1 g

Vanilla Egg Custard

Vegetarian

This is a recipe for a very gently set egg custard flavored with vanilla that is perfect for the Full Liquids stage of eating. It will keep well in the refrigerator for up to three days. A base of chopped fruit, like cherries, pears, peaches, or apricots, can be added in later stages of post-op eating to add texture and variety.

- 4 large eggs
- 1 (14-ounce) can light evaporated milk
- ⅔ cup low-fat milk
- 5 tablespoons Splenda granulated sweetener
- 2 teaspoons vanilla extract
- Ground nutmeg, for dusting (optional)

Preheat oven to 325°F.

In a medium bowl, beat the eggs with the evaporated milk, low-fat milk, sweetener, and vanilla. Strain and pour into seven heatproof ramekins or small custard cups. Dust the tops of the custards with ground nutmeg, if using.

Set the ramekins inside a heatproof baking dish and add hot water to come halfway up the sides of the ramekins.

Bake for 20 to 25 minutes, or until just set but still a bit wobbly.

Remove from the baking dish and allow to cool.

Refrigerate to chill before serving.

Serves 7

WLS portion ½ to 1

Calories per portion 135

Protein 9.3 g

Carbohydrate 9.8 g

Fat 6.4 g

4

STAGE 3: PUREED FOODS

Eating Well in Stage 3

If you don't experience any problems with the stage 2 Full Liquids regimen, then you will quickly move on to stage 3, which incorporates pureed foods.

This stage typically occurs 2 to 6 weeks after weight-loss surgery—although, once again, follow your bariatric team's advice on when to move on from a liquids regimen.

It's wise to start slowly and to make sure initially that your food choices are very soft and loose. First-stage baby food texture is what you are aiming for here. Even the softest pureed texture might need some extra "slack" from added fluid to make it the desirable consistency.

Progress to foods that can be easily crushed with a fork or mixed into a "slurry" with milk, gravy, or sauce. A small baby blender or mini-prep food processor can really help in these early days when portion sizes are small and the amount you can eat might well be the quantity that gets deposited on the sides of a larger processor or blender.

Don't be put off when something doesn't seem to suit you or taste right at this early stage—try it again a few days later. Oddly enough, some days something will go down easily and the next time it won't. Also learn to listen to your body and its signals of satisfaction and upset.

You will still need to be aiming for at least 2 quarts of liquids a day in addition to these small pureed meals. But now is the time to really enforce the **no-drink around mealtimes rule**: Don't drink for 30 minutes before and 30 minutes after (or during) a meal.

Aim for 4 to 6 small pureed meals per day. Remember to eat slowly, and as soon as you are full, *stop eating*! Just one extra teaspoon of food can send your newly replumbed system into overload, and—there is no pleasant way of saying this—what went down will come back up or make you feel very uncomfortable if you take too much on board. Remember, your new stomach pouch is only about the size of an egg.

You may now find it very convenient to freeze pureed foods in ice cube trays for this stage. You'll also be grateful for any that you stashed away pre-op. Meals in this form can be reheated quickly for serving, and variety is ensured rather than the relentless round of the same old dishes. Waste will also be reduced to a minimum. If you have a weight-loss surgery buddy, consider a trade of some of your dishes for his or hers to get extra variety at this stage.

This stage is akin to the "weaning" of a baby from milk to first solids. Very simple, bland purees with plenty of liquids are a good start, then gradually move to more flavorful options that have more texture but are still easy on the pouch, to finally textured purees with more "bite" and adventurous flavors. This is the stage at which you become friendly with the ramekin or custard cup for serving food.

Crispy foods that fall into bits in water, such as melba toast, crisp-breads, saltine crackers, and breadsticks, can also be introduced in the latter days of this stage 3. Chew them thoroughly until they are reduced to a smooth puree in your mouth. Don't mistake them for crunchy foods, like fruit and salad, which would cause problems at this stage.

Good Choices of Pureed Foods

- Mashed banana, with a little yogurt added, if desired
- Very soft and creamy scrambled egg
- Finely ground or pureed chicken or turkey in gravy
- Pureed fish in a thin sauce
- Pureed canned fish like sardines or tuna in a very thin sauce
- Plain low-fat cottage cheese
- Pureed mashed potato or mashed sweet potato with thin gravy
- Pureed canned and very tender cooked vegetables, such as carrot and cauliflower
- Low-fat and low-sugar fromage blanc
- Light and smooth low-fat and low-sugar mousse made with milk
- Warm mashed potato with low-fat cream cheese or other soft cheese
- Milk pudding, such as tapioca or sago, but keep the sugar to a minimum
- Pureed cooked cauliflower and cheese in a low-fat sauce, thinned with extra milk
- Pureed vegetable and chicken soups made with tender poultry pieces and soft vegetables
- Soft beans and lentils pureed to a smooth texture
- Pureed avocado
- Thick fruit smoothies, ideally homemade from fresh fruit and with no added sugar
- Low-sugar sorbets
- Silken or smooth tofu
- Crispy (not crunchy) foods like crispbreads, melba toast, saltine crackers, and breadsticks
- Soft and smooth low-fat pâté or spreads
- Finely textured low-fat and low-sugar salsas and dips

- Small portions of homemade soups, prepared vegetable and meat purees, and pureed main dishes that have been thinned with extra stock, milk, or gravy

In addition, take a daily multivitamin, calcium supplement, and any other supplement recommended or prescribed by your bariatric team.

Proper Tools

You will find getting into your new bariatric routine so much easier if you are prepared for the changes involved and get organized in advance. It really is crucial to stock up your pantry, refrigerator, and freezer (see page 23 in chapter 3), and it will also pay to invest in some kitchen gadgets to make your life a lot simpler once you return from your surgery. Together with the tried-and-tested recipes and the advice in this book, you will be all set.

You may be pleased to learn that nothing very expensive or special is required on a daily basis. However, there are a few small items that will keep things stress-free; these are worth investing in if you don't have them already.

Basic Kitchen Equipment

Kitchen Scale

A kitchen scale ensures that the quantities are correct and you're not guessing or eyeballing portion sizes. Modern digital scales can be easier to use and are often more accurate than mechanical scales.

Ice Cube Trays and Small Storage Containers

These are great for storing prepared soups and pureed meals. Simply make a batch of the food and pour it in, then freeze it until solid, pop it out, and transfer to a large freezer bag for long-term storage. It's a good idea to make some of these in advance of your surgery so that you have something to come home to. Most ice cube tray wells hold around 1 tablespoon of food, so you can remove 1 to 3 cubes depending on your current eating stage, keeping things nice and simple. A good selection of plastic or glass storage containers will also come in very handy. To save money here you could reuse yogurt tubs and other supermarket meal containers. Make sure you label everything to avoid any surprises!

Food Processor or Blender

This will be particularly valuable early on when you are in the liquid, pureed, and soft food stages. A processor will make short work of soups and smoothies. If you're going to buy a new blender, a small "baby" or single-portion-size one would be ideal as you will often be pureeing very small quantities of food.

Nonstick Cookware and Reusable Silicone Baking Sheets

Investing in these will keep you from using unnecessary amounts of oil or butter to stop food from sticking when you are broiling, baking, and roasting. Reusable silicone baking sheets are very hard-wearing, dishwasher-safe, and seem to last forever. They also save time on washing baked-on food off your cookware. You can buy the sheets in a roll so that you can cut them to size for different trays and dishes, or use ready-cut sheets.

A nonstick frying pan and skillet are also absolutely vital for making protein-filled omelets and dry-frying fish, chicken, and meat. You need only a spritz of low-fat nonstick cooking spray for a great result.

Small Ramekins

Little dishes like these are best for preparing and storing small meals. Microwave-friendly ones are perfect so you can cook and serve in one easy step.

Zip-Top Bags

These ingenious bags allow you to store foods in an airtight way in the freezer, cupboard, or refrigerator. Good-quality ones can be carefully washed and reused. You can also snip off the corner of one to make an instant piping bag.

Specialized Kitchen Equipment

There are countless kitchen gadgets around, but only those that are used repeatedly should earn a spot in the kitchen of a bariatric cook. These special ones are worth considering:

Air-Fryers

These machines made their name and gained their popularity due to the fact that they can give textural results similar to frying while using a minimum of oil. Notably, they cook fries that are crisp and golden with fat levels under 3 percent. They are therefore very good for making vegetable or sweet potato fries, which are lower in calories and fat than potato fries; stir-frying vegetables; cooking healthy cuts of lean fish, chicken, and meat without very much (if any) oil; roasting fruits for puddings; and even making risottos. They are such versatile machines. Some come with a rotating paddle for turning the food as it cooks; others have a fixed tray setup, which is ideal for those foods that crumble if repeatedly turned—but you may have to turn it over manually halfway through cooking.

Bento Lunch Box

This isn't essential but you may find it helpful for taking to work or if you are often out on the road during the day. It will enable you to keep your main meal, savory snacks, and sweet snacks in separate compartments. Packed with a freezer chiller pack, it also ensures food is kept cool and in good condition.

Electric Ice Cream Maker

These aren't as expensive as they used to be, and I find that ice creams, sorbets, and water ices made in a machine always have better, smoother textures than ones made by hand. Decide how often you are likely to use it before investing, but good bargains can be found at online auction sites.

Silicone Poach Pods and Soft Muffin Trays

These are real lifesavers for poaching eggs, baking frittatas, and making small cakes. Muffin trays are also ideal for holding the right size of savory dishes, like casseroles and stews, for storage. Freeze the food in the tray and then pop it out to store in a freezer bag when you are making large batches.

Mindful Eating

Have you started to recognize the difference between real hunger and imaginary hunger yet? It's critical as a weight-loss surgery patient to learn to eat with your head and not with your feelings. Emotional eating is destructive, so it's vital to look after yourself and learn to manage your feelings without involving food—which can be quite a task.

It's all too easy to mistake emotional hunger, like tiredness, stress, boredom, anger, or anxiety, for real hunger. So how can we stop ourselves from reaching for the cookie jar every time our day takes a turn for the worse?

First, check if you're really hungry. Ask yourself these questions:

- Is my stomach rumbling?
- Am I just thirsty?
- Is this a sudden attack of hunger or has it been steadily growing over the past few hours?
- Have I eaten in the last 3 to 4 hours?
- Is this a sudden urge to eat?
- Has my mood changed sharply?

If you answer yes to the final three questions, then it's more than likely that you are eating because you're hungry "for something" rather than physically hungry for food.

Now what? Here are six ways to stop eating for the wrong reasons:

1. Distract yourself with an activity. This could be anything you enjoy—reading, talking with a friend, gardening, going for a walk. It could be a pleasurable activity like planning a special vacation, or an emotional one like watching a sitcom on TV or looking through a favorite photo album. In fact, it can be absolutely anything that will take your mind off food and buy you some time.

2. Learn to self-soothe. When you reach to eat, ask yourself why. What else would make you feel better? Would it be better to have a soak in the bath or e-mail a friend? Learn to be mindful and choose food-free treats.

3. Teach yourself to spot triggers. Keeping a food diary can really help with this (see page 27). If you get into the habit of recording the situation, place, and company you are in when you find yourself wanting to eat, then you will start to understand what makes you tick and what people and events are your bariatric "enemies." Once you know that certain situations are a trigger, you can start to put some coping mechanisms in place to help you to deal with them.

4. Get into a regular eating pattern. It's not about being regimented, but it is crucial to have three meals a day at regular intervals, with perhaps a couple of small snacks in between. Please don't be tempted to skip meals—you need to eat in a regular pattern to learn the difference between real and imaginary hunger.

5. Choose food you love. You can only eat much smaller portions now, so it is important that you go for quality foods that you really enjoy. Eat slowly, really taste your food, and savor every bite. Make mealtimes into an event—sit down at a table, with cutlery, with no distractions like the TV.

6. Don't beat yourself up. Be kind to yourself and accept that the vast majority of people have emotions and issues around eating. This is the first crucial step toward improving your relationship with food.

Introducing Exercise

Even before you go in for your surgery, you will be advised to increase your activity levels in order to decrease your body fat and weight. It will also help you to make the transition to exercising more frequently after your operation.

In addition to changing the way you eat after surgery, you'll need to make sure you are moving more than you ever did before. Eating is only half the battle, and all health professionals agree that weight loss without exercise is slow and not as dramatic. If you want to see the best possible results, you must get moving!

Immediately after the surgery, you won't be able to exercise until you have fully recovered. But once you are given the all clear, you should make a slow but steady start, increasing your activity little by little. After about six weeks you should be able to manage a gentle workout.

People often ask, "What is the best exercise to do?" There's no right answer to this question. The best exercise is simply the one that you will stick to. There is no point in taking out an expensive gym membership if you don't enjoy going there. Thankfully, there are so many options—you will find one that suits your personality, wallet, and ability.

Walking is probably the best way to start—around the garden, up and down the stairs, around the neighborhood.

If you have difficulty walking or doing anything weight-bearing for any length of time, you should consider cycling on a stationary exercise bike or swimming. Aqua aerobics classes are also very good for weight-loss surgery patients (once all your wounds have healed).

Honey, I Shrunk Myself!

For enhanced weight loss and weight maintenance, the ball is now in your court. If you've never exercised before, here are some precautions to follow to make sure you're exercising safely:

- Start exercising *before* surgery, not just afterward.
- Take advice from your bariatric team—don't start exercising until they say you are ready.
- Begin with short walks—this will tone up your muscles and prepare your body for more strenuous activities.

- Do 5 to 15 minutes of cardio exercise before strength training. Strength training is what helps you to build muscle, but it's good to warm up the body with some cardio first.
- Start with 1 to 2 sets of 6 to 15 repetitions. Start small and build up gradually. Don't put your body under unnecessary stress in the early days as it will cause problems in the long run.
- Don't choose weights that are too heavy for you. It's important not to strain yourself. You should only feel a manageable amount of resistance.
- Keep a workout diary—this will keep you on track, help you monitor your progress, and motivate you.

For a fitter, healthier life, the best advice is to start by making small positive changes to your everyday activities that will soon make a big difference to your lifestyle:

- Take the stairs instead of the elevator.
- Park far away from the supermarket doors so you have to walk a bit farther when doing your shopping.
- Get off the bus one stop earlier and walk the rest of the way.
- Try walking or cycling instead of driving.
- Get a pedometer. Record your steps and try to increase by 10 percent each week, aiming eventually for 10,000 steps a day.
- Hide your TV remote and get up to change channels.
- Walk your dog daily.
- Walk up the steps on an escalator.
- Go up and down the stairs as much as possible during the day instead of stockpiling things at the bottom for carrying up all in one go.
- Get a yoga ball and sit on it when using the telephone or watching TV to master balance and improve core strength.
- View housework and gardening as a workout.

Recommended Exercise Types

- Aerobic—walking, dancing, swimming, cycling
- Non-weight-bearing—water-based activities, cycling on an exercise bike
- Resistance—free weights, machines, and exercise bands (These are all great for building strength. Ask a professional to show you how to use them correctly.)

Make sure that you rotate your workouts to avoid putting undue pressure on any joints.

How Often Should I Exercise?

You should be aiming for five 30-minute activity sessions every week. To start with, go for three 10-minute sessions and build from there. Be patient with yourself and don't set unrealistic targets.

Think of this as a long-term lifestyle change, not a fad that you will only stick with for a few months. Keep an exercise diary and stay focused—only you can make these changes, so be accountable.

Make exercise a top priority and you will soon start to accomplish your goals. It also helps to have an exercise buddy to support you and keep you on the straight and narrow.

The key is making it enjoyable, not a chore. But do check with your healthcare team before starting any exercise program, including walking.

Starting a Walking Program

Prior to surgery you will be advised to increase your activity levels to make the transition to exercising later more manageable, and to make the surgery easier by lowering your levels of body fat and weight. Then, after surgery, you'll be advised to increase your activity level, little by little, until you can manage a gentle workout.

But what kind of exercise? Gym memberships can be expensive; running or cycling outside can put stress on the body; swimming may be embarrassing if you're still very overweight; and opening hours of recreational fitness centers might not fit in with your working hours.

Walking is a great way to start. It's free, convenient, and easy on your body. Walking in short increments is also a great way to start toning up your muscles and preparing your body for future exercises. These are the reasons most bariatric teams recommend walking as the best form of exercise after weight-loss surgery.

So walking ticks all the boxes, but how do you get motivated to start and then maintain an active walking program?

- Make a commitment to yourself to walk come rain or shine. Don't let the weather be an excuse for not walking. If it's cold, then wrap up; raining, don a raincoat or take an umbrella; very hot, then apply sunscreen and take a sun hat and water.

- Plan ahead. Check your diary at the beginning of the week and decide and record which days you plan to walk. Then work your other chores and activities around these rather than the reverse. Don't let a busy life get in your way—make it work for you.

- Set a destination to reach. Knowing where you are heading often makes the time pass more quickly. Choose somewhere you want to visit—a shop, a friend's house, a library, or a beautiful spot. A reward will then come at the end of the walk.

- Change your destination frequently to keep things new and fun. Avoid routine and boredom by checking out new places that you may have promised to visit.

- Jazz up or calm down your walk as you wish. Some days you might want to walk listening to upbeat and energizing songs that will put extra pep in your step; other days you may just want to clear your mind and walk in solitude to mull over and channel your positive energy into plans and thoughts for the future. Do what suits you and your mood.

- Walk a dog—your own or a borrowed one. Dogs make wonderful walking companions and can be great motivators to stay active and up the ante on the length of your walking journey.

Breakfast and Lunch Ideas for Stage 3

Breakfast Ideas for Stage 3

- Any of the breakfast options listed for stage 2 (see page 29)
- Lightly scrambled or soft-cooked egg on whole-wheat toast
- Crackers with low-fat cheese spread
- Cornflakes or bran flakes saturated with low-fat milk
- Low-fat and low-sugar yogurt or fromage blanc with mashed banana
- Lightly cooked soft omelet
- Melba toast and low-fat cheese spread
- Very soft fruit compote without added sugar

Lunch Ideas for Stage 3

- Any of the lunch options listed for stage 2 (see page 29)
- 2 to 3 tablespoons fish with mashed potato and vegetables blended with a low-fat cheese sauce
- 2 to 3 tablespoons ground meat, casseroled meat, or curried meat with mashed potatoes or pasta, and vegetables blended with gravy or sauce
- 2 to 3 tablespoons cooked cauliflower and cheese blended with mashed potato
- 2 to 3 tablespoons dal blended with low-fat yogurt
- Small bowl of smooth or soft chunky soup blended with extra vegetables, cheese, or yogurt
- Wafer-thin meat and soft salad vegetables with low-fat dressing and breadsticks
- Baked beans on crispy toast
- Low-fat cream cheese or other soft cheese or pâté with crispbreads, tomato, and cucumber
- Poached or scrambled egg on toast

- Omelet with cheese or cooked vegetable filling
- Cottage cheese and crackers or crispbreads
- Couscous salad with meat, fish, or vegetables
- Low-fat hummus or other bean dip with melba toast or breadsticks

Pureed Foods Stage Recipes

- Beet and Butterbean Puree (page 57)
- Chickpea and Roasted Red Bell Pepper Puree (page 58)
- Leek, Pea, and Sweet Potato Puree (page 59)
- Sweet Roots Medley Puree (page 60)
- First Chicken and Vegetable Puree (page 61)
- Luscious Liver Special Puree (page 62)
- Fishy Dishy Salmon with Carrots and Tomato (page 63)
- Sweet Potato, Broccoli, and Pear Puree (page 64)
- Zesty Lemon Hummus (page 66)
- Fava Bean and Mint Dip (page 67)
- Chicken Liver Pâté (page 68)
- Tomato and Cilantro Salsa (page 69)
  - Variation: Salsa Rice (page 70)
- Masoor Dal (page 71)
- Easiest-Ever Spicy Tomato and Bean Soup (page 72)
- Gazpacho (page 73)
- Thai Chicken Soup (page 74)
- Warming Parsnip and Carrot Soup (page 76)
- Strawberry Hawaii Slush (page 77)
- Mango Lassi Dessert (page 78)
- Pumpkin Pie (page 79)

Beet and Butterbean Puree

Vegetarian

You can use virtually any canned bean in this puree mixture—cannellini, haricot, black-eyed peas, and the rest. Serve alone, with crackers, then finally with vegetable crudités when you can tolerate them.

- 1 (15-ounce) can butterbeans, drained and rinsed
- 1 garlic clove, crushed
- 1 tablespoon snipped fresh chives
- 1 tablespoon olive oil
- 1 tablespoon fat-free Greek yogurt
- Salt and freshly ground black pepper
- 1 (8-ounce) can beets in their juices, drained and chopped

Place the butterbeans, garlic, chives, olive oil, yogurt, and salt and pepper to taste in a food processor or blender and puree until smooth.

Add the beets and pulse to just incorporate, scraping down the sides of the food processor or blender once or twice as necessary.

Spoon into a serving bowl and chill until ready to serve.

Serves 4
WLS portion ½
Calories per portion 118

Protein 6 g
Carbohydrate 14.4 g
Fat 3.9 g

Chickpea and Roasted Red Bell Pepper Puree

Vegetarian

This puree is very easy to put together if you use bottled roasted red bell peppers. Choose the variety bottled in brine rather than in oil to avoid excess fat.

- 1 (14-ounce) can chickpeas, drained
- 2 bottled roasted red bell peppers, drained
- 2 garlic cloves, crushed
- ¼ cup tahini paste, preferably light roast
- Juice of 1 small lemon
- 2 tablespoons fat-free Greek yogurt
- ½ teaspoon red pepper flakes (optional)
- Salt and freshly ground black pepper

Place the chickpeas, roasted bell peppers, garlic, tahini, lemon juice, yogurt, red pepper flakes (if using), and salt and pepper to taste in a food processor or blender. Puree until smooth.

Spoon into a serving dish and chill until ready to serve.

Serves 4

WLS portion ½

Calories per portion 125

Protein 8.3 g

Carbohydrate 12.1 g

Fat 5.1 g

Leek, Pea, and Sweet Potato Puree

Vegan / Vegetarian / Suitable for Freezing

Sweet potatoes, with their naturally sweet taste and smooth texture, make a great early stage food. Here they are cooked with leeks and frozen peas for a puree that is full of nutrients. Choose the orange-fleshed variety of sweet potato when available since it is rich in beta-carotene as well as being a gorgeous color.

- 2 ounces leek, washed well and sliced crosswise
- 14 ounces sweet potato, peeled and chopped
- 1¼ cups vegetable stock
- Salt and freshly ground white pepper
- 2 ounces frozen peas

Place the leek, sweet potato, stock, and salt and white pepper to taste in a pan. Bring to a boil, reduce the heat to maintain a simmer, cover, and simmer for 15 minutes.

Add the peas and cook for 5 minutes more, or until the vegetables are very tender.

Puree in a blender or food processor until smooth or the desired consistency.

Let any leftover portions cool and then refrigerate them, or freeze them for later eating.

Serves 5

WLS portion 1

Calories per portion 75

Protein 1.8 g

Carbohydrate 16.6 g

Fat 0.6 g

Sweet Roots Medley Puree

Vegan / Vegetarian

Root vegetables like rutabaga, carrots, and parsnips make a nutritious puree for the very early days post-op. It's hard to judge quantities at this stage but aim initially for 1 to 2 tablespoons of puree and increase the quantity and thickness of the medley as time progresses.

- 4 ounces carrot, chopped
- 4 ounces potato, peeled and chopped
- 2 ounces parsnip, chopped
- 4 ounces rutabaga, chopped
- 1¼ cups low-fat milk (or water for vegans)
- Salt and freshly ground white pepper

Place all the vegetables, the milk, and salt and white pepper to taste in a saucepan. Bring to a boil, reduce the heat to maintain a simmer, cover, and simmer for 25 to 30 minutes until very tender.

Remove the vegetables with a slotted spoon and puree in a small blender or in a bowl using an immersion blender, adding as much cooking liquid as is necessary to reach the desired pureed consistency.

Let any leftover portions cool and then refrigerate them, or freeze them for later eating.

Serves 5

WLS portion 1

Calories per portion 53

Protein 2 g

Carbohydrate 11.2 g

Fat 0.3 g

TIP

If preferred, chopped butternut squash or pumpkin can be used instead of the potato.

First Chicken and Vegetable Puree

Suitable for Freezing

This is the ideal puree for reintroducing chicken to the menu. It's more like a chicken casserole mixture with the addition of peas. Puree until smooth to begin with, then process to a more textured consistency as you progress with recovery.

- 2 teaspoons low-fat spread or light butter
- 2 ounces leek, finely chopped
- 4 ounces skinless and boneless chicken breast, cut into chunks
- 3 ounces carrot, chopped

- 7 ounces sweet potato, peeled and chopped
- 2 sprigs fresh thyme
- 1 cup chicken stock
- Salt and freshly ground white pepper
- 2 ounces frozen peas

Melt the low-fat spread in a pan. Add the leek and cook until softened, about 5 minutes.

Add the chicken and cook for 3 to 4 minutes.

Add the carrot, sweet potato, thyme, stock, and salt and white pepper to taste. Bring to a boil, reduce the heat to maintain a simmer, cover, and simmer for about 15 minutes.

Add the peas and cook for 4 minutes more. Remove from the heat and remove and discard the thyme.

Place in a blender or food processor and puree until smooth or to the desired consistency.

Let any leftover portions cool and then refrigerate them, or freeze them for later eating.

Serves 4

WLS portion 1

Calories per portion 100

Protein 8.2 g

Carbohydrate 13 g

Fat 1.9 g

Luscious Liver Special Puree

Suitable for Freezing

It is always better to get your nourishment from food rather than supplements, and this liver and vegetable puree provides a hefty dose of iron, which is so vital for good health. Choose a light-flavored liver such as chicken, lamb, or calf rather than more robust pig liver for this dish.

- 6 ounces potato, peeled and chopped
- 1 teaspoon low-fat spread or light butter
- 1 teaspoon low-fat milk
- 3 ounces chicken, lamb, or calf liver
- 1 ounce leek, well washed and finely chopped
- 1 ounce mushrooms, finely chopped
- 2 ounces carrot, chopped
- ½ cup chicken stock
- Salt and freshly ground black pepper

Place the potato in a saucepan with enough water to cover and bring to a boil. Cook until tender, 10 to 15 minutes. Drain and mash with the low-fat spread and milk.

Meanwhile, trim the liver and chop it into pieces. In a medium saucepan over low heat, combine the liver, leek, mushrooms, carrot, stock, and salt and pepper to taste. Cook for about 8 minutes until cooked throught and tender. Remove from the heat.

Place the liver mixture in a blender or food processor and puree until smooth. Add the mashed potato and pulse a few times to mix with the liver puree.

Let any leftover portions cool and then refrigerate them, or freeze for later eating.

Serves 6

WLS portion 1

Calories per portion 66

Protein 4.7 g

Carbohydrate 9.5 g

Fat 1.1 g

Fishy Dishy Salmon with Carrots and Tomato
Vegetarian / Suitable for Freezing

This mixture of salmon with carrots, tomatoes, and just a sprinkling of cheese makes a creamy fish puree good for the early days of post-op eating. Blend the mixture to a very smooth puree or fork-mash it to a tender texture, depending on your stage of recovery.

- 8 ounces carrots, sliced crosswise
- 5 ounces skinned salmon fillet
- Low-fat milk
- 1 tablespoon low-fat spread or light butter
- 2 tomatoes, peeled, seeded, and chopped
- 1/3 cup grated low-fat hard cheese
- Salt and freshly ground white pepper

Bring a saucepan of water to a boil. Place the carrots in a steamer basket and steam over the boiling water for 15 to 20 minutes or until very tender. Set aside.

Meanwhile, place the salmon in a small pan, add enough milk to just cover, and simmer for about 4 minutes or until cooked through. Remove the salmon from the pan with a slotted spoon, reserving the cooking liquid, and set aside on a plate.

Melt the low-fat spread in a small pan, add the tomatoes, and cook until they are softened, about 5 minutes. Remove from the heat and stir in the cheese until melted, then add salt and white pepper to taste.

Place the tomato mixture in a blender or food processor with the cooked carrots and drained fish. Puree until smooth or to the desired consistency, adding some of the reserved cooking liquid, if necessary, to reach the desired consistency.

Let any leftover portions cool and then refrigerate them, or freeze for later eating.

Serves 4

WLS portion 1

Calories per portion 118

Protein 11.1 g

Carbohydrate 6.4 g

Fat 5.3 g

Sweet Potato, Broccoli, and Pear Puree

Vegan / Vegetarian / Suitable for Freezing

Most bariatrics find the pureed stage of eating postsurgery the most challenging, and it's easy to understand why. A dish that tastes wonderful when freshly cooked can taste very different when pureed or fork-mashed to within an inch of its life. Some retreat to the baby food aisle, only to be further disappointed. Well, here is a tasty and nutritional puree that is delightful and has an optional addition of dairy. The plain version is good, but the cheesy option has a stronger flavor and a better protein boost—the choice is yours.

- 1 (11-ounce) sweet potato, peeled and cut into chunks
- 1 small pear, peeled, quartered, and cored
- 4 ounces broccoli florets
- Salt and freshly ground black pepper
- 1 tablespoon low-fat milk (optional)
- ½ cup grated low-fat mature hard cheese (optional)

Bring a saucepan of water to a boil. Place the sweet potato, pear, and broccoli in a steamer basket and steam over the boiling water until each item is tender. The sweet potato will generally take longer (depending on the size of the chunks), so remove the pear and broccoli to the jar of a blender when they are cooked.

When tender, transfer the sweet potato to the blender with the pear and broccoli and add salt and pepper to taste. Puree until the desired consistency is reached. (Alternatively, mash the pear, broccoli, sweet potato, and salt and pepper to taste in a bowl until the desired consistency is reached.)

If desired, add the milk and cheese to the warm puree and stir until well combined and melted.

Serve at once or cool and freeze in small portions (an ice cube tray is ideal for this).

Serves 4

WLS portion 1

Calories per portion (with milk and cheese) 109

Protein 5.9 g

Carbohydrate 17.6 g

Fat 2.2 g

Zesty Lemon Hummus

Vegan / Vegetarian

A spoonful of hummus, or chickpea dip, makes a flavorsome mouthful during the Pureed Foods stage of eating after surgery. Later on, it makes a wonderful high-protein addition to vegetable crudités or a baked potato, or as a side dish for a broiled lamb steak. There are many commercial offerings available, but lots of them are laden with fat or additives, so it's better to make your own from scratch. It's a cinch in the blender or food processor.

- 1 (14-ounce) can chickpeas
- 2 tablespoons tahini paste
- 1 garlic clove, crushed

- Zest of 1 lemon
- Juice of 2 lemons
- Salt and freshly ground black pepper

Drain the chickpeas, rinse in cold water, and drain again thoroughly.

Place in a blender or food processor with the tahini paste, garlic, lemon juice, lemon zest, and salt and pepper. Puree on high power until smooth.

Spoon into a small serving dish, cover, and refrigerate to chill before serving.

Serves 4

WLS portion ½

Calories per portion 115

Protein 5.8 g

Carbohydrate 9.1 g

Fat 6.2 g

Fava Bean and Mint Dip

Vegetarian

This is a tasty dip to have with a few breadsticks or simply to eat by the small spoonful during the Pureed Foods stage. Remember to remove the skins from the beans; otherwise the dip will not be as smooth as your stomach pouch might like.

- 2 cups shelled young fava beans
- Generous ¾ cup fat-free Greek yogurt
- Small handful fresh mint leaves
- 1½ tablespoons grated Parmesan
- ½ garlic clove, crushed
- Salt and freshly ground white pepper
- Crisp breadsticks, for serving

Bring a saucepan of water to a boil. Cook the fava beans for about 8 minutes, or until very tender. Drain and rinse under cold water. When cool enough to handle, rub off and discard the skins.

Place the skinned fava beans, yogurt, mint, Parmesan, garlic, and salt and pepper to taste in a blender or food processor and puree until smooth.

Serve lightly chilled with crisp breadsticks for dipping, if desired.

Serves 4

WLS portion ½

Calories per portion (without breadsticks) 80

Protein 8.1 g

Carbohydrate 7 g

Fat 2.1 g

Chicken Liver Pâté

This is a very healthy version of a traditional chicken liver pâté, made smooth and creamy with the addition of fat-free fromage blanc instead of the usual cream. It's great to eat with a crispbread, or with vegetable crudités at later stages. The low-fat spread or light butter pour-over coating isn't essential. but if you plan to store for it more than one day, the coating ensures the pâté stays moist and doesn't dry out in the refrigerator. It can, of course, be discarded from any WLS portion.

- 1 tablespoon low-fat spread or light butter
- 1 red onion, finely chopped
- 1 garlic clove, crushed
- 8 ounces chicken livers, washed and trimmed
- 2 teaspoons tomato paste
- Salt and freshly ground black pepper
- 2 tablespoons fat-free fromage blanc

For the topping

- 4 tablespoons low-fat spread or light butter, melted
- Bay leaves, for garnish (optional)

Heat the low-fat spread in a nonstick skillet. Add the onion and garlic and cook over low heat for about 5 minutes, until softened.

Add the chicken livers and cook for 5 to 8 minutes more, until they are cooked through and no longer pink. Add the tomato paste and salt and pepper to taste, mixing well.

Place the mixture in a blender or food processor with the fromage blanc and puree until smooth. Transfer to a serving dish, cover with plastic wrap, and chill for at least 2 hours.

To make the topping: Pour a little melted low-fat spread over the pâté to seal in moisture. To garnish, add a couple of bay leaves to the topping before it sets, if desired.

Serves 4

WLS portion ½ to ¾

Calories per portion (without topping) 95

Protein 12.7 g

Carbohydrate 4.4 g

Fat 2.9 g

Tomato and Cilantro Salsa

Vegan / Vegetarian

A spoonful of salsa can lift the ordinary dish into something celebratory and may be just the flavorsome mouthful you desire in the Pureed Foods stage of eating. A small drizzle or dollop of this fresh herby salsa on a cracker might just hit the spot when other foods don't. Later in your weight-loss surgery journey, it makes a welcome side dish to a steamed or baked fish fillet, a grilled chicken breast, or a broiled slice of halloumi cheese, or a great topping for a bariatric-friendly pizza. Keep a batch in the refrigerator and see how versatile it is.

- 2 large tomatoes
- 3 garlic cloves, crushed
- 2 tablespoons lime juice
- 2 tablespoons chopped cilantro leaves
- 1 teaspoon chopped fresh chili (optional)
- ½ teaspoon ground cumin
- Salt and freshly ground black pepper

Remove the skins from the tomatoes if not tolerated. Place the tomatoes in a food processor with the garlic, lime juice, cilantro, chili (if using), cumin, and salt and pepper to taste. Process in bursts, for either a chunky or smooth-textured salsa as preferred.

Alternatively, finely chop the tomatoes and garlic and combine them in a bowl with the lime juice, cilantro, chili (if using), cumin, and salt and pepper to taste.

Chill until needed but bring to room temperature for serving.

Serves 4

WLS portion ½

Calories per portion 26

Protein 1 g

Carbohydrate 4.4 g

Fat 0.4 g

continued ▶

TIP
Salsa Rice

Any brown or basmati rice is delicious when mixed with salsa. Simply stir 2 tablespoons salsa into ½ cup cooked rice for a main meal accompaniment or rice salad dish.

Masoor Dal

Vegan / Vegetarian / Suitable for Freezing

Here is a recipe for a lentil-based dal that is perfect for the Pureed Foods stage of eating after bariatric surgery. This is reasonably well spiced and hits the spot after many bland foods. If you don't like your food too spicy, then halve the spices in the recipe below.

- Low-fat nonstick cooking spray
- 1 teaspoon fenugreek seeds
- 1 onion, finely chopped
- 1 teaspoon ground cumin
- 1½ teaspoons garam masala
- 1 teaspoon ground coriander
- 1 teaspoon turmeric
- 1 small red chili pepper, seeded and finely chopped
- 2 garlic cloves, chopped
- 1¾ cups dry red lentils
- 5 cups vegetable stock
- Handful of fresh cilantro leaves, chopped
- Salt and freshly ground black pepper

Generously spritz a large saucepan with cooking spray. Heat the pan over medium heat, then add the fenugreek seeds and gently toast in the pan for 2 minutes.

Add the onion, cumin, garam masala, coriander, turmeric, chili, and garlic and cook for 2 minutes more, stirring occasionally.

Add the lentils and stock, bring to a boil, then reduce the heat to maintain a simmer and cook for 20 to 30 minutes more, until thick and soup-like.

Add the fresh cilantro and salt and pepper to taste. Mix well.

Transfer to a blender and puree, or leave the dal chunky for a little more texture. Serve warm.

Serves 8

WLS portion ½

Calories per portion 165

Protein 11.4 g

Carbohydrate 27.5 g

Fat 1.6 g

Easiest-Ever Spicy Tomato and Bean Soup

Vegan (without yogurt) / Vegetarian / Suitable for Freezing

It may well be that in the early days after surgery you don't feel like cooking but have a hankering for a homemade soup. This one may fit the bill because it is very quickly made with some kitchen-cupboard ingredients that have all the prep work done for you. Puree the soup for early stage eating but leave chunky, if preferred, later down the line.

- Low-fat nonstick cooking spray
- 1 onion, finely chopped
- 2 celery stalks, finely chopped
- 1 garlic clove, crushed
- 2 teaspoons mixed dried herbs
- 1 teaspoon red pepper flakes (optional)
- 1 (14-ounce) can chopped tomatoes
- 1 (14-ounce) can low-sodium, reduced-sugar baked beans in tomato sauce
- 2½ cups vegetable stock
- Salt and freshly ground black pepper
- 4 tablespoons fat-free Greek yogurt (optional)

Generously spritz a large saucepan with cooking spray. Heat the pan over medium heat, add the onion, celery, garlic, herbs, and red pepper flakes (if using), and cook for 5 minutes.

Add the tomatoes, baked beans, stock, and salt and pepper to taste. Mix well. Bring to a boil, reduce the heat to maintain a simmer, cover, and simmer for 25 minutes.

Puree the soup in a blender or food processor until smooth, or leave chunky, as desired.

Serve in warmed bowls with 1 tablespoon of the yogurt swirled on top of each portion, if desired.

Serves 4

WLS portion ½

Calories per portion 135

Protein 8.9 g

Carbohydrate 20.3 g

Fat 1.2 g

Gazpacho

Vegan / Vegetarian

This is a refreshing cold soup that can be served chunky or smooth, so it's perfect for the Pureed Foods stage of eating and beyond. At later stages of eating, consider serving it with croutons, chopped olives, diced cucumber, and hard-boiled eggs to add interest and in some cases additional protein.

- 2 slices brown or whole-wheat bread, cut into small cubes
- 2½ cups tomato juice
- 2 garlic cloves, crushed
- ½ cucumber, peeled, seeded, and finely chopped
- 1 green bell pepper, cored, seeded, and finely chopped
- 1 red bell pepper, cored, seeded, and finely chopped
- 1 large mild Spanish onion, finely chopped
- 1½ pounds tomatoes, peeled, seeded, and finely chopped
- 1 to 2 tablespoons red wine vinegar
- 2 tablespoons olive oil (optional)
- 2 tablespoons chopped fresh mixed herbs
- Salt and freshly ground black pepper

Place the bread cubes in a bowl and pour over the tomato juice. Leave to soak for 5 minutes, then squeeze the bread to extract the juice. For a smooth pureed soup, place the bread cubes in a blender and reserve the juice. For a chunky version, place the cubes and tomato juice in a large bowl without pureeing.

For a smooth pureed soup, add the garlic, cucumber, bell peppers, onion, and tomatoes to the blender and puree until smooth. Add the reserved tomato juice, vinegar to taste, oil (if using), herbs, and salt and black pepper to taste. Mix well. Alternatively, for a chunky version, add the vegetables and seasonings to the bread and tomato juice in the bowl and mix well.

Chill for at least 1 hour before serving.

SERVES 4

WLS portion ½ to ¾

Calories per portion (without oil) 150

Protein 6.2 g

Carbohydrate 29.4 g

Fat 1.5 g

Thai Chicken Soup
Suitable for Freezing

Just when you're tiring of bland purees and "safe-tasting" soups, along comes this flavor popper! It's a chicken soup zipped up with Thai seasonings and enriched and thickened with vegetables. It has been made here using reduced-fat coconut milk, which does have a tendency to split a little during cooking, but has a better nutritional profile than full-fat coconut milk for bariatrics. Choose whichever you wish. Serve pureed or chunky according to your stage of eating.

- 1 (14-ounce) can reduced-fat coconut milk
- 1 large onion, finely chopped
- 1 garlic clove, crushed
- 1 tablespoon chopped peeled fresh ginger
- 1 teaspoon chopped fresh chili
- 1 teaspoon tom yum paste or other Thai curry paste
- 2½ cups chicken stock
- 8 ounces skinless and boneless chicken, chopped
- 8 ounces mixed chopped vegetables (carrots, cauliflower, green beans, and leeks, for example)
- Salt and freshly ground white pepper
- Chopped fresh cilantro, for garnish (optional)

In a large saucepan, combine the coconut milk, onion, garlic, ginger, chili, and tom yum paste and mix well.

Set the pan over high heat. Add the stock, mix well, and bring to a boil. Reduce the heat to maintain a simmer and cook, uncovered, for 20 minutes.

Add the chicken, vegetables, and salt and white pepper to taste. Cover and simmer for 1 hour.

Puree in a blender or food processor until smooth, or leave chunky for later-stage eating.

Spoon into warmed bowls and garnish with chopped cilantro, if desired, to serve.

Serves 4

WLS portion ⅓ to ½

Calories per portion 130

Protein 15.7 g

Carbohydrate 7.6 g

Fat 4.1 g

Warming Parsnip and Carrot Soup

Vegan / Vegetarian / Suitable for Freezing

Here is a "comfort blanket" soup made from parsnips and carrots flavored with curry-esque spices and orange. It's a thrifty recipe and well worth making in bulk since it freezes well.

- Low-fat nonstick cooking spray
- 1 onion, chopped
- 1 small red chili, seeded and chopped
- 1 tablespoon garam masala
- 1 pound parsnips, chopped
- 1 pound carrots, chopped
- 4¼ cups hot vegetable stock
- Scant 1 cup water
- Zest and juice of 1 orange
- Salt and freshly ground white pepper

Generously spritz a large saucepan with cooking spray. Heat the pan over medium heat, add the onion and chili, and cook for 5 minutes until softened. Add the garam masala and cook for 1 minute more.

Add the parsnips, carrots, stock, and water. Bring to a boil, reduce the heat to maintain a simmer, cover, and simmer gently for 20 to 25 minutes, until the vegetables are very tender.

Using an immersion blender, puree the mixture until smooth, or transfer to a blender or food processor and puree.

Stir in the orange zest, orange juice, and salt and white pepper to taste. Reheat gently, then ladle into warmed bowls to serve.

Serves 4

WLS portion ½

Calories per portion 185

Protein 4.8 g

Carbohydrate 35 g

Fat 3 g

Strawberry Hawaii Slush

Vegan / Vegetarian

This is a delicious, healthy, pureed beverage that you can drink morning, noon, or night in the very early stages after weight-loss surgery. For convenience, prepare the fruit in advance and keep it in the freezer to make as needed.

- 1 cup sliced strawberries
- 1 ripe banana, peeled and cut into chunks
- 1 ripe mango, pitted, peeled, and cubed
- 1 ripe peach, pitted, peeled, and sliced
- 1 small slice watermelon, rind and seeds removed, chopped
- ½ cup fresh orange juice or 100% orange juice
- 1 tablespoon lemon juice

Place the strawberries, banana, mango, peach, and watermelon on a plastic tray or a tray covered with nonstick parchment paper and freeze until solid, about 2 hours.

Transfer the frozen fruit to a food processor or blender, add the orange juice and lemon juice, and puree until smooth.

Pour into glasses to serve.

Serves 2

WLS portion ½ to 1

Calories per portion 170

Protein 2.3 g

Carbohydrate 39.1 g

Fat 0.7 g

Mango Lassi Dessert

Vegetarian

This is a creamy and refreshing dessert-type dish that is based on lassi, a chilled yogurt drink popular in India. Serve very cold for a sweet treat or as the perfect end to a spicy meal.

- 2 whole cardamom pods
- 2 ripe mangoes, pitted, peeled, and roughly chopped
- 8 ounces fat-free Greek yogurt
- Finely grated zest and juice of ½ lime
- 1½ teaspoons filtered honey
- 1 ounce dried mango, cut into strips (optional)

Chill 3 medium serving glasses. Remove the cardamom seeds from the pods and crush them to a fine powder using a pestle and mortar.

Puree the mango flesh in a food processor or blender until smooth. Fold in the yogurt, lime zest, lime juice, crushed cardamom seeds, and honey.

Spoon into the chilled glasses and serve decorated with strips of dried mango, if desired.

Serves 3

WLS portion ½

Calories per portion (without dried mango) 138

Protein 8.6 g

Carbohydrate 26.4 g

Fat 0.3 g

Pumpkin Pie

Vegetarian

This is a recipe for traditional pumpkin pie but without the added sugar. Ideally it is made crust-free for the Pureed Foods stage of eating, but if you wish to serve it in a homemade or premade graham cracker crumb shell, see the tip at the bottom of the recipe.

- 1 (15-ounce) can pure pumpkin
- ½ cup Splenda granulated sweetener
- 1 teaspoon ground cinnamon
- ½ teaspoon ground ginger
- ¼ teaspoon ground cloves
- Dash of salt
- 2 large eggs
- 1 (12-ounce) can light evaporated milk
- Sugar-free whipped cream, for serving (optional)

Preheat oven to 300°F.

In a large bowl, mix the pumpkin with the sweetener, cinnamon, ginger, cloves, and salt. Beat in the eggs, one at a time, until well blended. Stir in the evaporated milk and mix well.

Pour the pumpkin mixture into a deep 9-inch glass pie plate and bake for 30 to 35 minutes, until set but still a little wobbly in the center.

Remove from the oven and allow to cool to room temperature. Serve warm, or cool and then refrigerate until serving. Cut into wedges and serve topped with a little sugar-free whipped cream, if desired.

Serves 6

WLS portion ½

Calories per portion 132

Protein 8.2 g

Carbohydrate 14.4 g

Fat 5.1 g

TIP

The uncooked pumpkin mixture can be poured into a premade pastry or graham cracker crumb shell and then baked in a preheated 350°F oven for 30 to 35 minutes. (Remember that this will affect the nutritional value of the dish.)

5

STAGE 4: SOFT FOODS

Eating Well in Stage 4

There's a very fine line between those foods that are considered pureed in stage 3 and those that are categorized as soft in stage 4. Usually, soft foods have more of an identifiable appearance to their natural state (for example, a carrot may be whole and identified as such but very tender in stage 4, rather than pureed to a paste-like appearance as in stage 3), but both are still soft enough to be easily digested by the newly replumbed bariatric digestive system.

Dishes cooked for this stage are not tremendously different from those found in stage 5—the ones you will cook and eat for the rest of your life—except that they have most likely been cooked longer for increased tenderness or selected for their soft texture.

Initially, these foods will be tender enough to be pureed in a blender or food processor or even mashed with a fork, but as time progresses, they will take on more of a bite or resistance and look much chunkier in appearance. This is the final stage to complete before you can progress to stage 5, or pretty much what everyone else is eating: healthy food for life.

This is definitely the stage at which you should be preparing and cooking your own recipes from scratch (if you haven't been too enthusiastic about it before). That way you know exactly what you're eating. Many processed foods and ready-made dishes have hidden sugars and fats (not to mention salt) added to make them taste good, which can be the proverbial banana skin for the weight-loss surgery patient.

Try a few simple recipes to start with and certainly become vigilant about reading and deciphering the nutritional information on the packaged foods you're eating. You're aiming for a low-fat regimen (as a guideline, look for foods with less than 5 g of fat per 100 g). As for sugar, people's toleration levels vary enormously, but try not to venture beyond the 7 to 10 g sugar hit per portion for reasonably safe eating without trouble.

During this stage, you will still need to keep your fluids up in addition to your normal regimen of three meals (and possibly two small snacks). Again, **remember the rule of not drinking before, during, and just after eating** (as for stage 3).

This is also the time to be a little more adventurous. Try reintroducing pasta, rice, bread, and those foods you've avoided so far. You may sail through their reintroduction without problems, but if you do find that they don't sit comfortably, take a break and try them again later. Don't assume these foods are off the menu for life—you may well just not be ready for them, or you may have to try cooking them in a different way for success.

Likewise, salad and crunchy-type foods can be tried—just remember to chew, chew, and chew some more when eating them so that they can gradually become part of your new dietary program. Those salad vegetables and fruits with skins might be the most tricky, so peel them or remove the skins first.

Try to have three small meals per day on a small salad or side plate with perhaps a couple of healthy snacks throughout the day, if needed.

Good Choices for Soft Foods

- Tender casseroles, curries, and stews of a thinnish consistency
- Very gently cooked and soft omelet, plain or filled with a tender filling
- Poached or soft-cooked egg
- Soft beans, lentils, and peas, mashed, if desired
- Small portions of home-cooked or ready-prepared main dishes like cottage pie, shepherd's pie, fish in sauce, mild chili, pasta Bolognese, and vegetable hot pots
- Cooked pasta, rice, and polenta with sauce
- Yogurts, fools, and mousses containing soft pieces of fruit
- Slow-cooker main-meal favorites that are cooked until meltingly tender
- Porridge and bircher-style soaked muesli with tender pieces of dried or softened fruit
- Spanish omelet (*tortilla*)
- Low-fat and low-sugar cheesecake
- Lentil and soft veggie burgers

In addition, take a daily multivitamin, calcium supplement, and any other supplements recommended or prescribed by your bariatric team.

Slow Down . . .

Eating too fast is a very common problem among people who are overweight. When you gobble your food down too quickly, your body isn't given the time to recognize its natural "full" signals, which means that you end up eating too much and then feel uncomfortable—as if you are going to pop.

Eating too much food postsurgery is very dangerous, so you must train yourself to eat more slowly and break this nasty habit.

Here are a few strategies that can help:

- Eat with a set of cutlery (i.e., a knife and a fork, not just a fork or a spoon). Put both utensils down between each bite and chew slowly about 20 times. Count to 60 or watch the second hand on a clock rotate for 60 seconds before taking your next mouthful. Savor the flavor and texture of your food. Be mindful about what you are eating.
- Sit down to eat, ideally at a table rather than on the sofa. Don't watch TV, read, or drive while eating. There is a tendency to eat faster when you are distracted or trying to do something else at the same time.
- Watch the clock. Try to make your meal last for 20 minutes. This is important because it takes your stomach 15 to 20 minutes to send a signal to the brain to say you are full and don't need to eat any more.
- Using a child's set of cutlery or a pair of chopsticks can also help to slow you down. Alternatively, if you are right-handed, try eating with your left hand, and vice versa. The awkwardness will slow down your pace and should mean that you aren't the first person to finish eating your meal.
- You might recognize that other members of your family eat too fast without realizing you too are guilty. Try eating in front of a mirror to gauge how fast you are eating and how big your bites really are. It could be an eye-opener.
- Finally, before you start to eat your meal, pause to take a breather for a minute or so. During this time, commit yourself to eating slowly and mindfully. There is no rush, and as soon as you teach yourself this lesson, you will find that you start to recognize the feeling of being full a lot more quickly. And when you do—stop eating right away and don't push it!

Weighing Things Up

There is a huge temptation to jump on the scale every morning, or even more often, after weight-loss surgery. The number you see can dictate your day. Up, down, or just the same as yesterday, those numbers can determine how you're going to feel for the rest of the day: defeated and down, or happy and victorious. It's a ritual that results in an ongoing mental battle.

But ask yourself this: *Is that number really a good reflection of me?* The truth is that the scale is not a great way to measure your success when it comes to weight loss and body change.

Why not? Well, the scale doesn't measure what your body is made of (it can't differentiate between fat, muscle, and water). It doesn't measure if you're losing fat or losing muscle—it simply records loss of pounds and ounces (so you could be losing weight, but is it the right kind and from the right place?). The scale doesn't tell you what's going on in your body and how to address it, nor does it address what's going on in your head—nor, come to think of it, does it accurately record whether or not you're on track in relation to your current needs.

So why do we let such a poor system take up so much of our time and energy? It's a ritual—a regimen, a habit. Well, it's time to change this. So many bariatric teams recommend that you *ditch the scale* between surgery and hospital appointments (where they will accurately record your weight on reliable and tested equipment), and replace weighing yourself with something that will more accurately measure your progress at home: Take your measurements the old-fashioned way with a tape measure. Record your chest, waist, hip, dominant arm, dominant leg, neck, and any other measurement every month and note the differences.

Look in the mirror and see how your clothes are fitting. Are they getting baggier? If you're losing fat and toning up, then you will lose inches and it will show in the fit of your clothes even if it doesn't register on the scales.

Check to see if your shape changes. Taking a regular photograph of yourself in the same position can highlight this. Losing fat often means you change shape, not just change size.

Consider some other medical numbers that can act as a barometer for how well things are going. What's your blood pressure like? Your cholesterol level? Your blood sugar level compared to last month? How's your thyroid? These are better indicators of your current situation and more important than your numbers in terms of weight for long-term health.

Have your medication levels changed? Have you been able to reduce or cut out your pills and potions altogether? Again, these have much more "weight" than those numbers on the scale when it comes to measuring wellness.

The challenge is to break this bad habit if you have it, or resist the urge in the first place, and stop stepping on the scales too frequently. Once a week is recommended and more than enough between appointments with your bariatric team. Adopt some of the above tips instead; they will measure your progress better and more accurately reflect your well-being.

Hair Today . . . Gone Tomorrow?

Hair loss and thinning after bariatric surgery is common regardless of the type of weight-loss surgery procedure. Often this is mild but sometimes can be more severe.

There are several reasons why people lose hair after weight-loss surgery. Some hair loss can be expected and attributed to any form of surgery that involves anesthesia—it's a commonly experienced side effect—but here's the main reason why and how it works.

At any given time about 90 percent of your hair is in a "growing phase" and the remaining 10 percent is in a "resting phase." After the hair rests for 2 to 3 months, it falls out and new hair grows in to replace it. Anesthesia causes more hair to go into this resting phase than normal, more like 30 percent. So it follows that 2 to 3 months after surgery, this larger-than-usual amount of hair falls out. This is usually temporary and the hair does replenish itself in time.

However, there are additional reasons for hair loss after weight-loss surgery that relate more to rapid weight loss and malabsorption of nutrients in the body. It is this rapid loss of weight and reduced nutrition that can cause additional hair loss and hair thinning. Any kind of rapid weight loss will produce hair loss (it doesn't only happen with surgery), and a lack of nutrients can compound the effect. So it goes without saying that the best way to minimize this loss is to maximize nutrition.

After weight-loss surgery, patients need to aim for about 70 g of protein a day for good nutrition and to supplement their diet with a daily multivitamin. This is essential for all patients but especially important for gastric bypass patients whose "replumbing" means their body cannot absorb all the nutrients it takes in as food. Your bariatric team may also recommend a daily dose of calcium citrate, an additional B vitamin complex tablet, and an iron supplement; follow their guidelines to the letter.

It's not easy to get a high level of protein in your diet in the early days after weight–loss surgery when appetite and toleration levels of food are low. Some people who constantly underscore in achieving the recommended levels opt to drink a protein drink supplement. There are many kinds available in a multitude of flavors, but if you're considering one, check out its nutritional profile and choose one that is low in fat, sugar, and calories. Don't opt for the body-builder's version!

Others boost their protein levels by adding dried skimmed milk or unflavored protein powder to their food. Tasteless and virtually unnoticeable, it can be stirred into soups, stews, smoothie-type drinks, and most pureed foods for an invisible but welcome protein boost.

Focusing on getting the correct nutrition is the best way to minimize hair loss and maximize hair regrowth after surgery. Most hair loss happens about 3 to 4 months after surgery, but hair growth cycles do go back to normal after about 1 year. Gentle shampoos and some hair supplements may also help, but there is no guaranteed over-the-counter solution.

Emergency Measures: Build Your Own "Bariatric 911" Box

When you are following a bariatric eating plan, it can be all too easy to fall off the wagon—for instance, when plans change at the last minute or you get stuck in traffic and can only find fast food to eat. Being prepared can stop these instances from becoming a problem. Why not keep an emergency supply of "bariatric 911" foods in the trunk of your car or office desk drawer so that you're never stranded? They can sometimes be a lifesaver.

Here are some good choices:

- Low-fat and low-sugar cereal bars
- Small packet of unsalted nuts
- Small jar of low-fat pâté or paste in an airtight sealed jar with crackers (don't forget a small knife for spreading)
- Low-fat and low-sugar protein drink (ideally ready to drink)
- Rich tea cookies or light graham crackers

- Small bag of mixed seeds
- Small package of olives
- Healthy low-fat and low-GI snack or meal pot
- Small packet of dried fruit
- Stay-fresh container of bariatric-friendly cereal and a couple of mini cartons of long-life low-fat milk
- Small bag of soy nuts
- Small package of beef jerky (keep an eye on the sell-by date)
- A couple of sugar-free candies or mints
- Low-fat snacks like oatcakes, rice cakes, rye crispbread, or melba toast

Breakfast and Lunch Ideas

Breakfast Ideas for Stage 4 (Same as Stage 3)

- Any of the breakfast options listed for stage 2 (see page 29)
- Lightly scrambled or soft-cooked egg on whole-wheat toast
- Crackers with low-fat cheese spread
- Cornflakes or bran flakes saturated with low-fat milk
- Low-fat and low-sugar yogurt or fromage blanc with mashed banana
- Lightly cooked soft omelet
- Melba toast and low-fat cheese spread
- Very soft fruit compote without added sugar

Lunch Ideas for Stage 4 (Same as Stage 3)

- Any of the lunch options listed for stage 2 (see page 29)
- 2 to 3 tablespoons fish with mashed potato and vegetables blended with a low-fat cheese sauce
- 2 to 3 tablespoons ground meat, casseroled meat, or curried meat with mashed potato or pasta and vegetables blended with gravy or sauce
- 2 to 3 tablespoons cooked cauliflower and cheese blended with mashed potato
- 2 to 3 tablespoons dal blended with low-fat yogurt
- Small bowl of smooth or soft chunky soup blended with extra vegetables, cheese, or yogurt
- Wafer-thin meat and soft salad vegetables with low-fat dressing and breadsticks
- Baked beans on crispy toast
- Low-fat cream cheese or other soft cheese or pâté with crispbreads, tomato, and cucumber
- Poached or scrambled egg on toast

- Omelet with cheese or cooked vegetable filling
- Cottage cheese and crackers or crispbreads
- Couscous salad with meat, fish, or vegetables
- Low-fat hummus or other bean dip with melba toast or breadsticks

Soft Foods Stage Recipes

- Turkey Bolognese (page 93)
- Cottage Pie (page 94)
- Bean and Sausage Cassoulet (page 96)
- Herder's Pie (page 98)
- Beef Patitsada (page 100)
- Lamb Tagine (page 101)
- Fruity Spiced Pork (page 103)
- Pasta Bake with Beets and Smoked Ham (page 105)
- Smoked Salmon, Cucumber, and Dill Pâté (page 107)
- Cheesy Polenta with Barbecue Shrimp (page 108)
- Simplest Fisherman's Pie (page 110)
- Cod en Papillote with Pesto and Cherry Tomatoes (page 111)
- Easy Vegetarian Chili (page 112)
- French-Style Lentils with Eggs (page 114)
- Three-Cheese Egg Bake (page 115)
- Spinach, Chickpea, and Tomato Curry (page 116)
- One-Dish Vegetable Hot Pot (page 117)
- Vegetable Fried Wild and Basmati Rice (page 118)
- Chinese Fried "Rice" with a Difference (page 119)
- Speedy Lentil Burgers (page 121)
- Apple Bircher Muesli (page 123)
- Porridge with Apple, Cinnamon, and Pecans (page 124)
- Greek Yogurt with Honey, Berries, and Seeds (page 125)
- Strawberry Soufflé Omelet (page 126)
- Creamy Lemon Blueberries (page 127)

Turkey Bolognese
Suitable for Freezing

All over Italy, every family has its own favorite Bolognese recipe, many of them handed down over generations. Served with pasta, it is staple fare and usually made with beef or a mixture of pork and beef. This version is particularly bariatric-friendly because it uses ground turkey, which is high in protein and lower in saturated fat than ground beef—but is just as full of flavor.

- Low-fat nonstick cooking spray
- 1 large onion, finely chopped
- 1 pound lean ground turkey
- 1 garlic clove, crushed
- 2 carrots, finely chopped
- 1 (14-ounce) can chopped tomatoes
- 2 tablespoons tomato paste
- Generous 1 cup water or light stock
- ½ teaspoon dried oregano
- 1 tablespoon Worcestershire sauce
- Salt and freshly ground black pepper
- Cooked pasta, for serving

Generously spritz a large nonstick pan with cooking spray. Heat the pan over low heat, add the onion, and cook for 2 to 3 minutes to soften.

Raise the heat to medium high, add the ground turkey, and cook for 1 to 2 minutes, stirring and breaking up any lumps.

Add the garlic, carrots, chopped tomatoes, tomato paste, water, oregano, Worcestershire sauce, and salt and pepper to taste. Bring to a boil, reduce the heat to maintain a simmer, cover, and simmer for 45 to 50 minutes, until cooked through and tender.

Serve hot with a little freshly cooked pasta.

Serves 4

WLS portion ½

Calories per portion (without pasta) 256

Protein 32.3 g

Carbohydrate 10.8 g

Fat 9.4 g

Cottage Pie

Suitable for Freezing

Cottage pie is a British staple made with ground meat and vegetables. It doesn't really matter which kind of ground meat you use, although this version with ground turkey works well because it is low in fat. When cooked, the pie produces a pouch-friendly protein layer of tender, moist meat topped with a comforting layer of mash. The recipe below uses regular potatoes, but you could use sweet potato, carrot, rutabaga, or a mixture—whatever pleases your palate and pouch.

- Low-fat nonstick cooking spray
- 1 onion, chopped
- 1 leek, well washed and chopped
- 1 carrot, chopped
- 1 pound lean ground turkey
- 1 tablespoon Worcestershire sauce
- 1 (14-ounce) can chopped tomatoes
- 4 ounces frozen peas
- 1 tablespoon tomato paste
- 1 teaspoon chopped fresh thyme
- Salt and freshly ground black pepper
- 2¼ pounds potatoes, peeled and chopped into small pieces
- 2 tablespoons fat-free yogurt
- ¼ cup grated low-fat cheese

Preheat oven to 400°F.

Generously spritz a pan with cooking spray. Heat the pan over low heat, add the onion, leek, and carrot and cook for 10 minutes. Remove from the pan and set aside.

Generously spritz the pan again with cooking spray, add the turkey, and cook for 5 minutes. Add the vegetable mixture, Worcestershire sauce, chopped tomatoes, peas, tomato paste, thyme, and salt and pepper to taste. Cook for 20 minutes until tender, then transfer to an ovenproof dish.

Meanwhile, place the potatoes in a saucepan with enough water to cover and bring to a boil. Cook until tender, 15 to 20 minutes, then drain the potatoes and mash with the yogurt and salt and pepper to taste. Spoon the mashed potatoes over the meat mixture and sprinkle with the cheese.

Bake for 30 minutes until golden. Serve hot.

Serves 4

WLS portion ½

Calories per portion 398

Protein 31.3 g

Carbohydrate 50 g

Fat 9.2 g

Bean and Sausage Cassoulet

Suitable for Freezing

This hearty meat dish includes mixed beans and looks rustic and home-cooked enough to pass for a long-labored specialty—without the effort. It doesn't need anything more than a light salad accompaniment.

- Low-fat nonstick cooking spray
- 4 reduced-fat or high-meat-content chipolata sausages (or other long, skinny, link-style sausages), weighing about 8 ounces total
- 1 large onion, sliced
- 14 ounces skinless and boneless chicken breasts, cut into bite-size pieces
- 1 teaspoon smoked paprika
- 2 (14-ounce) cans chopped tomatoes
- Salt and freshly ground black pepper
- 1 (15-ounce) can mixed beans in tomato sauce
- ½ ounce fresh oregano leaves, chopped

Generously spritz a large, deep, nonstick sauté pan or skillet with cooking spray. Heat over medium heat, add the sausages, and cook for 3 to 4 minutes until lightly browned on all sides.

Remove the sausages from the pan with a slotted spoon and set aside.

Spritz the pan again with cooking spray, add the onion, chicken, and paprika, and cook for 4 to 5 minutes until the chicken is browned and the onion has softened.

Return the sausages to the pan and add the tomatoes and salt and pepper to taste. Bring to a boil, reduce the heat to maintain a simmer, cover, and simmer for 30 minutes, stirring occasionally, until the chicken is very tender and cooked through.

Add the mixed beans and half of the oregano, mixing well. Cook, uncovered, for 10 minutes more, until the beans are heated through and the sauce has thickened.

Serve hot, sprinkled with the remaining oregano.

Serves 4

WLS portion ½

Calories per portion 355

Protein 39.1 g

Carbohydrate 30.7 g

Fat 7.4 g

Herder's Pie

Suitable for Freezing

This is a ground beef and bean pie with a topping that has a hefty portion of soft rutabaga instead of all potato. Rutabaga is considered easier to digest by bariatrics and using some in place of potato brings down the calorie and carb content of the dish. However, it's a pie that is hearty enough to satiate nonbariatric, "man-size" appetites, so it's ideal for the whole family. Serve with seasonal vegetables alongside.

- 1¾ pounds lean ground beef
- 1 large onion, finely chopped
- 2 large carrots, chopped
- 1¼ cups passata or smooth crushed tomatoes
- 1 beef bouillon cube, crumbled
- 3 tablespoons Worcestershire sauce
- Salt and freshly ground black pepper
- 1½ pounds rutabaga, chopped
- 4 large potatoes, peeled and chopped
- 1 (15-ounce) can low-sugar baked beans in tomato sauce
- ¼ cup grated low-fat cheese (optional)

Preheat oven to 300°F.

In a nonstick ovenproof pan set over moderate heat, brown the ground beef. Drain off any excess fat in the pan, then add the onion and carrots and cook for 5 to 10 minutes more, until the vegetables are softened.

Add the passata, bouillon cube, Worcestershire sauce, and salt and pepper to taste, mixing well. Cook for 5 minutes.

Cover and bake for 1 hour. Remove from the oven and raise the oven temperature to 400°F.

Meanwhile, bring a saucepan of water to a boil. Add the rutabaga and cook until soft, then drain and mash to a puree. At the same time, place the potatoes in a saucepan with enough water to cover and bring to a boil. Cook the potatoes until tender, then drain and mash to a puree. Mix the rutabaga puree with the mashed potatoes until well combined.

Stir the beans into the beef mixture and spoon into one large or six individual baking dishes. Top evenly with the mashed rutabaga and potato mixture. Sprinkle with the grated cheese (if using) and bake for 20 to 25 minutes until browned. Serve hot.

Serves 6

WLS portion ½

Calories per portion 394

Protein 35.8 g

Carbohydrate 48.2 g

Fat 6.2 g

Beef Pastitsada
Suitable for Freezing

This slow-cooked beef, flavored with allspice and red wine, comes from the Greek island of Corfu. It's ideal if you're having a crowd over for supper—just pop it in the oven and forget about it until you're ready to eat. Weight-loss surgery patients may find this is one of the first ways they can eat beef again (other than ground beef), since it is gentle on the new stomach pouch. Serve with rice or soft pureed potato, if you can tolerate a little, plus some seasonal green vegetables.

- Low-fat nonstick cooking spray
- 1 pound lean beef round, cut into bite-size pieces
- 12 shallots, peeled
- 4 ounces baby carrots, trimmed
- 1 teaspoon ground allspice
- ¾ cup red wine
- 1 (14-ounce) can chopped tomatoes with garlic (or plain, if preferred)
- ⅔ cup beef stock
- Salt and freshly ground black pepper

Preheat oven to 300°F.

Generously spritz an ovenproof sauté or casserole pan with cooking spray. Add half the beef and cook over a high heat for about 5 minutes, until well browned. Transfer to a plate and set aside. Drain any excess fat from the pan. Repeat with the remaining beef.

Add the shallots to the pan and stir-fry for 2 to 3 minutes or until just starting to color.

Return the beef to the pan and add the carrots, allspice, wine, tomatoes, stock, and salt and pepper to taste, mixing well.

Cover and bake for 3½ hours, or until tender and the juices are rich and thick. Serve with rice or potatoes and seasonal green vegetables.

Serves 4
WLS portion ½
Calories per portion 240

Protein 30.8 g
Carbohydrate 9.8 g
Fat 6.4 g

Lamb Tagine

Suitable for Freezing

Tagine is the name for the distinctive-shaped cooking pot found everywhere in Morocco, where this dish is most popular. You can, of course, just use a casserole dish with a tight-fitting lid to cook this very tender and flavorful stew. It is typically served with couscous.

- 1 teaspoon ground ginger
- 1 teaspoon ground coriander
- 1 teaspoon turmeric
- Low-fat nonstick cooking spray
- 1 pound diced lean lamb
- 1 onion, chopped
- 3 garlic cloves, crushed
- 2 large carrots, chopped
- 1 (14-ounce) can chopped tomatoes
- 2/3 cup soft dried apricots, halved
- 1¼ cups vegetable stock
- 2 tablespoons soy sauce
- Salt and freshly ground black pepper
- Cooked couscous, for serving (optional)

Preheat oven to 300°F.

Mix the ginger with the coriander and turmeric in a dish. Add the lamb and toss to mix. Leave to marinate for at least 30 minutes.

Generously spritz a large nonstick pan with cooking spray. Heat the pan over high heat, add the lamb in batches, and sauté until browned. Transfer to a tagine or casserole dish.

Reduce the heat to medium, add the onion, and cook gently for 5 minutes. Add the garlic and carrots and cook for 2 minutes more.

continued ▶

Add the tomatoes, apricots, stock, soy sauce, and salt and pepper to taste. Bring to a boil, pour over the lamb, cover, and bake for about 2 hours, until very tender.

Serve with couscous, if desired.

Serves 4

WLS portion ½

Calories per portion (without couscous) 285

Protein 34.4 g

Carbohydrate 23.8 g

Fat 5.8 g

Fruity Spiced Pork

Suitable for Freezing

Here's a recipe for a tender, slow-cooked pork casserole. It has a fruity and spicy flavor from the addition of dates, apricots, and mellow spices like cinnamon and mace. You could serve it with simple mashed potatoes, a baked potato, rice, or couscous—whatever strikes your fancy that you can tolerate. If you like a casserole with a thicker finished consistency, then just add a little cornstarch dissolved in water toward the end of the cooking time.

- Low-fat nonstick cooking spray
- 1¾ pounds stewing pork or pork leg, cut into bite-size pieces
- 1 large onion, sliced
- 3 stalks celery, sliced
- 2 garlic cloves, chopped
- 1 teaspoon ground cinnamon
- 1 teaspoon ground mace or freshly grated nutmeg
- 1 teaspoon mild curry powder
- 2 tablespoons chopped fresh thyme leaves
- ⅔ cup chopped soft dried dates
- ⅔ cup chopped soft dried apricots
- Juice of 1 orange
- 2 cups white wine or vegetable stock
- Salt and freshly ground black pepper cornstarch, dissolved in water to form a slurry (optional)
- ¼ cup walnut pieces
- 2 tablespoons chopped fresh parsley

Preheat oven to 325°F.

Generously spritz a large nonstick skillet with cooking spray. Heat over moderate heat, add the pork in batches, and cook on all sides until browned. Using a slotted spoon, transfer the pork to an ovenproof casserole dish, reserving the juices in the pan.

Add the onion, celery, garlic, cinnamon, mace, and curry powder to the pan juices and cook for 3 to 4 minutes, stirring frequently.

continued ▶

Add the thyme, dates, apricots, orange juice, wine, and salt and pepper to taste. Bring to a boil, then pour the mixture over the pork. Cover and transfer to the oven. Bake for 1½ to 2 hours, until the pork is very tender. If desired, stir in the cornstarch slurry toward the end of the cooking time to thicken the sauce in the casserole.

Dry-fry the walnut pieces in a small skillet over medium high heat until lightly browned. Sprinkle the nuts and chopped parsley over the casserole and serve.

Serves 6

WLS portion ½

Calories per portion 265

Protein 29.6 g

Carbohydrate 25.6 g

Fat 5 g

TIP
Slow-Cooker Method

Prepare the pork as above but reduce the wine or stock to 1¼ cups. Place the browned pork and vegetable-fruit mixture in a slow-cooker. Cover and cook on high for 1 hour. Reduce the cooker setting to low and cook for 3 to 4 hours more, until the pork is very tender. Finish for serving as above.

Pasta Bake with Beets and Smoked Ham

I know many bariatrics who struggle with pasta and an equal number who don't. If you can tolerate pasta, this tender mix of whole-wheat pasta with beets, ham, and vegetables is wonderfully warming and filling. It doesn't need anything more than a simple salad accompaniment.

- 3 cups whole-wheat dried pasta shapes (such as penne)
- 4 tablespoons low-fat spread or light butter
- 1 onion, chopped
- 1 garlic clove, crushed
- 2 tablespoons all-purpose flour
- 1½ cups low-fat milk
- 1½ cups grated low-fat hard cheese
- 1 cup shredded smoked ham
- ¼ cup snipped fresh chives
- Salt and freshly ground black pepper
- 1 pound cooked beets, chopped

Preheat oven to 350°F.

Bring a large pot of salted water to a boil. Cook the pasta according to the package instructions, drain, and reserve.

Melt the low-fat spread in a heavy-bottomed pan set over low heat. Add the onion and garlic and cook until softened, 10 to 15 minutes.

Whisk in the flour, then gradually add the milk, whisking constantly to break up any lumps. Raise the heat to high and bring to a boil, then reduce the heat slightly and simmer steadily for 2 to 3 minutes to cook the flour.

Reduce the heat to low, add half the cheese, and stir to melt it into the sauce. Add the ham, chives, and salt and pepper to taste, mixing well.

continued ▶

Stir in the cooked pasta and beets, then spoon the mixture into a large baking dish. Scatter the remaining ¾ cup cheese over the top and bake for 20 minutes, until golden brown and bubbly.

Allow to stand for 5 minutes before serving.

Serves 6

WLS portion ½

Calories per portion 405

Protein 27.3 g

Carbohydrate 63.6 g

Fat 5.1 g

Smoked Salmon, Cucumber, and Dill Pâté

Here is a deliciously creamy and soft pâté or spread that is ideal for wraps, as a topping for crackers, or as an accompaniment to crunchy vegetable crudités as soon as you can tolerate them.

- 6 ounces smoked Alaskan salmon
- 1¾ cups fat-free cream cheese or other soft cheese
- 2 tablespoons chopped fresh dill
- Finely grated zest of 1 lemon
- 1 tablespoon lemon juice
- ¼ cucumber, peeled, seeded, and finely chopped
- Freshly ground white pepper
- Sprigs of fresh dill, for garnish (optional)

Chop half of the smoked salmon into small pieces and slice the remainder into strips.

Mix the cream cheese with the dill, lemon zest, lemon juice, cucumber, and white pepper to taste. Fold in the chopped smoked salmon and place the mixture in a serving dish.

Top with the remaining salmon strips and garnish with a few sprigs of fresh dill, if desired. Serve lightly chilled.

Serves 4

WLS portion ⅓ to ½

Calories per portion 185

Protein 19.4 g

Carbohydrate 5.1 g

Fat 9.3 g

Cheesy Polenta with Barbecue Shrimp

Vegan / Vegetarian / Suitable for Freezing

Polenta might well be the comforting soft food that you desire after weight-loss surgery. This cheesy variation is wonderful alone, without any additions, in the very early days. It does, however, taste sensational when topped with a barbecue shrimp mixture. You can buy low-sugar barbecue sauce, but the easy-to-make, bariatric-friendly version in the tip at the end of this recipe works very well. Try it—you'll find a multitude of uses for this tangy sauce.

For the polenta
- 2¼ cups water
- 4½ ounces dry instant polenta
- ¼ cup low-fat milk
- 2 tablespoons grated Parmesan

For the shrimp
- Low-fat nonstick cooking spray
- 1 large red onion, finely chopped
- 2 scallions, finely chopped
- 2 carrots, cut into thin julienne strips
- 1 red bell pepper, cored, seeded, and finely sliced
- ½ teaspoon sweet paprika
- 1 cup fresh or canned chopped tomatoes (with their juices)
- 1 pound shrimp, peeled
- ¼ cup low-sugar barbecue sauce
- Salt and freshly ground white pepper

To prepare the polenta: Bring the water to a boil in a large saucepan. Add the polenta and cook for 3 minutes. Add the milk and Parmesan, stirring well. Cover and keep warm.

To prepare the shrimp: Generously spritz a large skillet with cooking spray. Heat over medium heat, add the red onion, scallions, and carrots, and cook for 2 minutes.

Add the bell pepper and paprika and cook for 2 minutes more.

Add the tomatoes with their juices and the peeled shrimp. Cover and cook for 2 to 3 minutes, until the shrimp are cooked and tender.

Stir the barbecue sauce into the shrimp and cook for 1 minute more. Season with salt and white pepper.

To serve, check the polenta and add a little more boiling water if it seems too thick.

Spoon the polenta onto warmed serving plates and top with the barbecue shrimp mixture. Serve at once.

Serves 4

WLS portion ½

Calories per portion 310

Protein 34.4 g

Carbohydrate 35 g

Fat 4 g

TIP

Homemade Barbecue Sauce

- Cooking spray
- 1 onion, finely chopped
- 1 garlic clove, crushed
- 5 ounces double-concentrated tomato paste
- 1 (12-ounce) can Diet Coke or Diet Pepsi

- 1/3 cup low-sugar tomato ketchup
- 1 tablespoon Dijon mustard
- 1 tablespoon Worcestershire sauce
- 1 teaspoon smoked paprika
- Salt and pepper

Generously spritz a pan with cooking spray. Heat over medium heat, add the onion and garlic, and cook for 4 to 5 minutes until softened. Add the tomato paste, diet soda, ketchup, mustard, Worcestershire sauce, and paprika, and season with salt and pepper. Bring to a boil, reduce the heat to maintain a simmer, and simmer for 15 minutes until cooked and thickened.

Makes 10 servings

WLS portion ½ to 1

Calories per portion 23

Protein 1.1 g

Carbohydrate 4.1 g

Fat 0.3 g

Simplest Fisherman's Pie

Suitable for Freezing

This favorite has been given a bariatric makeover to produce a comforting dish that supplies nourishment with nurture. Make in a large dish for family-style eating or small individual dishes (like ramekins) for single-dish serving. Stash a few servings in the freezer for those days when you don't feel like cooking from scratch. Serve with seasonal vegetables alongside.

- 3 pounds potatoes, peeled and chopped
- 4 ounces fat-free Greek yogurt
- Salt and freshly ground white pepper
- 1 pound assorted fresh and smoked skinless and boneless fish, cut into bite-size pieces
- ⅔ cup shelled raw shrimp
- ¾ cup fat-free cream cheese or other soft cheese
- Juice of 1 lemon
- 3 tablespoons snipped fresh chives

Place the potatoes in a saucepan with enough water to cover and bring to a boil. Cook until tender, 15 to 20 minutes. Drain the potatoes and mash with the yogurt and salt and white pepper to taste.

Preheat oven to 350°F.

Place the fish and shrimp in a large ovenproof dish or divide evenly among 6 small heatproof baking dishes. Dot with the cream cheese and sprinkle with the lemon juice, chives, and salt and pepper to taste.

Spread the mashed potatoes over the fish mixture and bake for 45 to 50 minutes until the fish and shrimp are cooked through and the mashed potatoes are golden.

Serve hot.

Serves 6

WLS portion ½ to ¾

Calories per portion 350

Protein 25.9 g

Carbohydrate 44.1 g

Fat 8.1 g

Cod en Papillote with Pesto and Cherry Tomatoes

If you're looking for a complete low-fat meal that virtually cooks itself, then here is the perfect recipe. It features cod fillet topped with a little pesto and a few cherry tomatoes and baked in its own foil parcel to succulent tenderness. Slip the tomatoes from their skins after cooking but before eating if you have a problem with digesting them.

- Low-fat nonstick cooking spray
- 4 (5-ounce) frozen cod fillets
- 2 teaspoons pesto sauce
- Juice of 1 lemon
- 4 small bunches cherry tomatoes
- Salt and freshly ground white pepper

Preheat oven to 375°F.

Cut four sheets of aluminum foil and spritz with cooking spray, ensuring that they are large enough to wrap the fish fillets and their topping.

Place a frozen cod fillet on top of each piece of foil. Spread each fillet with ½ teaspoon of the pesto sauce and sprinkle with lemon juice. Top each with a small bunch of cherry tomatoes and salt and pepper to taste. Spritz again with cooking spray. Fold the foil around the fish to create a packet and place on a baking sheet.

Bake for 25 to 30 minutes or until the fish and tomatoes are cooked through and tender.

Serve in their foil packets, removing any skins and stalks from the tomatoes before eating.

Serves 4

WLS portion ½

Calories per portion 150

Protein 27.9 g

Carbohydrate 2.6 g

Fat 2.9 g

Easy Vegetarian Chili

Vegan / Vegetarian / Suitable for Freezing

Nothing could be easier to prepare and have on the table in next to no time than this vegetable chili. The recipe, packed full of goodness, uses canned kidney beans in a mild chili sauce, but if you want a chili with a bit more heat, add a chopped red chili pepper with the vegetables. Any leftover chili makes a good omelet filling.

- Low-fat nonstick cooking spray
- 1 onion, sliced
- 2 red bell peppers, cored, seeded, and cut into bite-size chunks
- 1 tablespoon mild chili powder
- 1 large carrot, cut into bite-size chunks
- 2 medium sweet potatoes, peeled and cut into bite-size chunks
- 1 (14-ounce) can chopped tomatoes with garlic
- 1 cup vegetable stock
- 1 zucchini, cut into bite-size chunks
- 1 (14-ounce) can kidney beans in chili sauce
- 2 ounces haricots verts, trimmed and halved
- Cooked rice, for serving

Generously spritz a large nonstick pan with cooking spray. Heat over medium heat, add the onion, and cook for 5 minutes until softened.

Add the bell peppers and cook for 2 minutes more. Add the chili powder and cook for 1 minute, stirring constantly.

Stir in the carrot, potatoes, tomatoes, and stock and simmer for 15 to 20 minutes.

Add the zucchini and the kidney beans with their sauce and simmer for 5 minutes more.

Finally, add the haricots verts and simmer for 5 to 10 minutes, or until all the vegetables are tender.

Serve hot over rice, if tolerated and desired.

Serves 6

WLS portion ½ to ¾

Calories per portion (without rice) 130

Protein (without rice) 7.8 g

Carbohydrate (without rice) 13.5 g

Fat (without rice) 5 g

French-Style Lentils with Eggs

Vegetarian

This is one of those kitchen-cupboard and refrigerator standbys that fits the bill on so many occasions. It's great for brunch on the weekend, provides a quickly cooked midweek family supper, and makes a fail-safe tender and flavorful dish for the Soft Foods stage of eating.

- Low-fat nonstick cooking spray
- 1 small onion, finely chopped
- 1 small carrot, finely chopped
- 1 celery stalk, finely chopped (optional)
- Generous ½ cup dry Puy lentils
- 1 teaspoon tomato paste
- 1¾ cups hot vegetable stock
- ½ (14-ounce) can chopped tomatoes
- 2 sprigs fresh thyme
- Salt and freshly ground black pepper
- ¼ Savoy cabbage, finely shredded
- 2 large eggs

Generously spritz a pan with cooking spray. Heat over low heat, add the onion, carrot, and celery (if using), and cook for 10 to 15 minutes until soft.

Add the lentils, tomato paste, stock, tomatoes, thyme, and salt and pepper to taste, mixing well. Bring to a simmer and cook for 15 minutes. Stir in the cabbage and continue to cook for 5 minutes, or until the cabbage is tender.

Meanwhile, bring a large pan of water to a boil. Add the eggs and cook for 7 minutes. Shell and halve or quarter the eggs.

Divide the lentils between two warmed dishes, then top each with one cut-up egg to serve.

Serves 2

WLS portion ½

Calories per portion 340

Protein 24.9 g

Carbohydrate 41.2 g

Fat 5.8 g

Three-Cheese Egg Bake

Vegetarian

This recipes scores on so many levels: It's soft and pouch-friendly; is versatile enough to be served for breakfast, lunch, or supper; has a huge amount of protein; can be served hot, warm, or cold; and tastes fantastic. It's bound to become a bariatric and family favorite.

- Low-fat nonstick cooking spray
- 6 large eggs
- ¼ cup all-purpose flour
- 1 teaspoon baking powder
- Salt and freshly ground white pepper
- 1 tablespoon snipped fresh chives
- 1 cup low-fat milk
- 1 cup low-fat cottage cheese
- 4 ounces low-fat cream cheese or other soft cheese, cubed
- 1 cup chopped low-fat sharp-flavored hard cheese
- 2 tomatoes, sliced (optional)

Preheat oven to 350°F.

Generously spritz a deep 7 x 9–inch baking dish (or similar-size dish) with cooking spray.

In a large bowl, beat the eggs with the flour, baking powder, and salt and white pepper to taste. Stir in the chives.

Add the milk, cottage cheese, cream cheese, and hard cheese, mixing well. Don't worry if the mixture looks lumpy at this stage; it will cook to a smooth, soft, creamy consistency.

Pour the mixture into the prepared dish and top with the sliced tomatoes (if using).

Bake for 35 to 45 minutes, or until well-risen and golden but still wobbly in the center. Remove from the oven and allow to stand for about 15 minutes before serving while warm. Alternatively, allow to cool and refrigerate until ready to serve.

Serves 4
WLS portion ½
Calories per portion 290

Protein 31.4 g
Carbohydrate 14.2 g
Fat 12.4 g

Spinach, Chickpea, and Tomato Curry

Vegan (with yogurt) / Vegetarian

This is a lightly spiced low-fat vegetarian curry dish that can be easily and quickly made from mostly kitchen pantry items. Serve with a little naan, if you can tolerate it, for an Indian-style meal.

- Low-fat nonstick cooking spray
- 1 garlic clove, chopped
- 1 small onion, finely chopped
- 2 tablespoons chopped peeled fresh ginger
- 1 tablespoon medium curry paste (Mughlai blend works well)
- 1 (14-ounce) can chopped tomatoes
- 1 (14-ounce) can chickpeas, undrained
- Salt and freshly ground black pepper
- 8 ounces fresh spinach, washed and shredded
- 4 tablespoons fat-free Greek yogurt (optional)
- 4 tablespoons chopped fresh cilantro leaves

Generously spritz a medium pan with cooking spray. Heat until hot, add the garlic, onion, and ginger, and cook until softened and golden. Stir in the curry paste and cook for 1 minute.

Add the tomatoes and simmer, stirring occasionally, for 5 minutes to make a thick sauce.

Stir in the chickpeas with their liquid and salt and pepper to taste. Bring to the boil. Reduce the heat to maintain a simmer and simmer for 10 minutes.

Add the spinach and cook gently for 2 minutes or until the spinach is just tender and cooked.

Serve each portion topped with a tablespoon each of the yogurt (if using) and the cilantro.

Serves 4

WLS portion ½

Calories per portion 135

Protein 9.2 g

Carbohydrate 17.2 g

Fat 3.4 g

One-Dish Vegetable Hot Pot

Vegan / Vegetarian

This is a simple hot pot that can be cooked and on the table in 35 minutes. If you want an especially tender result for the early stages of post-op eating, cook the dish for an additional 10 minutes. It is good with cooked quinoa but equally tasty with roasted garlic flatbread. The pesto is an optional ingredient, but the dish is all the better for its addition.

- Low-fat nonstick cooking spray
- 2 leeks, well washed and sliced
- 4 ounces baby carrots
- 1 small rutabaga, chopped
- 1 garlic clove, finely chopped
- 2¼ cups vegetable stock
- Salt and freshly ground black pepper
- 4 ounces spring greens or cabbage, shredded
- 1 (14-ounce) can borlotti beans or other beans, drained
- 2 tablespoons pesto (optional)

Generously spritz a large pan with cooking spray. Heat over low heat until hot, add the leeks, carrots, rutabaga, and garlic, and cook for 10 minutes until the vegetables are soft and golden.

Add the stock and salt and pepper to taste, then cover and simmer for 10 to 15 minutes, or until the vegetables are tender.

Add the spring greens or cabbage and the drained beans. Cover and simmer for 5 minutes more, until piping hot and cooked through.

Stir in the pesto (if using) and serve at once.

Serves 4

WLS portion ½

Calories per portion (with pesto) 140

Protein 8.1 g

Carbohydrate 15.3 g

Fat 5 g

Vegetable Fried Wild and Basmati Rice

Vegetarian

Some bariatrics have trouble digesting rice after surgery and others sail through without problems. If you can eat rice, this dish of tender wild and basmati rice cooked with vegetables, herbs, and a lightly scrambled egg mixture makes a great supper. It's also great cold as a packed lunch.

- ¾ cup wild and basmati rice mix
- Low-fat nonstick cooking spray
- 1 red onion, chopped
- 1 red bell pepper, cored, seeded, and chopped
- 1 zucchini, sliced crosswise
- 1 garlic clove, crushed
- 4 ounces baby cherry tomatoes, halved
- 4 large eggs
- Salt and freshly ground black pepper
- 2 tablespoons chopped fresh basil leaves

Cook the rice mix according to the package instructions until tender. Drain and keep warm.

Meanwhile, generously spritz a large skillet or frying pan with cooking spray. Heat over high heat, add the onion, bell pepper, zucchini, and garlic, and cook until tender and golden, 4 to 5 minutes.

Add the tomatoes and cook for 1 to 2 minutes more, until soft and tender. Remove from the pan with a slotted spoon and keep warm.

Beat the eggs with salt and black pepper to taste, then pour into the skillet and cook, stirring constantly until lightly scrambled.

Mix the warm rice with the cooked vegetables, cooked eggs, basil, and salt and black pepper to taste. Serve while still warm.

Serves 4

WLS portion ½

Calories per portion 285

Protein 13.5 g

Carbohydrate 41.4 g

Fat 7.2 g

Chinese Fried "Rice" with a Difference

The difference? No rice! This is a dish made with cauliflower that is prepared to look, and many say taste, like fried rice in all its Chinese-takeout glory. If your pouch can't tolerate rice post-op, it may well be very happy with this substitute. You will need to use a microwave to prepare the cauliflower for this recipe.

- 1 cauliflower, trimmed and cut into florets
- Low-fat nonstick cooking spray
- 2 large eggs, beaten
- Salt and freshly ground black pepper
- 2 garlic cloves, crushed
- 2 teaspoons finely chopped peeled fresh ginger

- 1 small red chili, seeded and finely chopped
- 1 onion, finely chopped
- 4 ounces cooked ham, bacon, or pork, cut into thin strips
- 2/3 cup shelled cooked shrimp
- 2 tablespoons light soy sauce
- 4 scallions, sliced
- 1 cup bean sprouts

Place the cauliflower in a microwave-proof dish and microwave on full power for 4 to 5 minutes, depending on wattage. Do not add any water. Place in a food processor and pulse until the cauliflower resembles grains of rice.

Generously spritz a large sauté pan or wok with cooking spray. Heat over medium-high heat, add the eggs and salt and pepper to taste, and cook for about 1 minute, stirring, until lightly scrambled. Remove the eggs, chop, and set aside.

Generously spritz the pan again, add the garlic, ginger, chili, and onion, and cook for 1 to 2 minutes. Add the ham and cook until golden.

Add the shrimp and cauliflower "rice" and toss well to mix.

continued ▶

Add the chopped eggs with the soy sauce, most of the scallions, and the bean sprouts. Stir-fry until well heated through, 2 to 3 minutes. Sprinkle with the remaining scallions and serve at once.

Serves 4

WLS portion ½

Calories per portion 165

Protein 19.8 g

Carbohydrate 9.1 g

Fat 5.5 g

Speedy Lentil Burgers

Vegetarian

These burgers are just the thing to make if you have some leftover cooked lentils but can also be made using packaged precooked lentils. Many come already seasoned with salt, pepper, herbs, and spices so be judicious when adding more seasoning. Serve in a lettuce leaf wrap (rather like a breadless bun) if you want to eat the burger bun-style, and top with a yogurt and mint (or other herb) dip (see page 166), if desired.

- 1 cup cooked lentils
- 1 scallion, very finely chopped
- 2 tablespoons chickpea flour (garbanzo bean flour)
- 1 egg, beaten
- ¼ cup grated Parmesan
- ½ teaspoon dried mixed herbs
- Salt and freshly ground black pepper
- Low-fat nonstick cooking spray
- Yogurt dip (see page 166), for serving (optional)
- Lettuce leaves, for serving (optional)

Mix the lentils with the scallion, flour, egg, Parmesan, herbs, and salt and pepper to taste, mixing well.

Divide the lentil mixture into 4 portions and shape them into small patties or burgers on a board with the aid of a circular cookie cutter or ring mold.

Generously spritz a large skillet with cooking spray. Heat over medium heat, then use a spatula to transfer the patties to the pan and cook until golden on the underside, about 5 minutes.

Carefully flip the burgers with the spatula, reduce the heat to low, and cook for 2 to 3 minutes more, until golden on all sides.

continued ▶

Serve warm, topped with a little yogurt dip and wrapped in lettuce leaves, if desired.

Serves 2   *Protein 13.5 g*

WLS portion 1   *Carbohydrate 14.1 g*

Calories per portion (without   *Fat 8.2 g*
dip) 185

Apple Bircher Muesli

Vegetarian

This deliciously fresh and nutrient-rich breakfast dish can be eaten right away or prepared and soaked overnight for an even creamier and softer texture.

- 2⅓ cups old-fashioned rolled oats
- Generous ¾ cup unsweetened soy milk
- ½ cup unsweetened apple juice
- 3 tablespoons fat-free Greek yogurt
- 1 tablespoon filtered honey
- Juice of ½ lemon
- 2 dessert apples (such as Ginger Gold or Gala), peeled, cored, and grated (for a very soft texture) or finely chopped
- ½ cup fresh blueberries

In a mixing bowl, combine the oats, soy milk, and apple juice, mixing well. Leave to stand overnight if a very soft creamy texture is preferred.

Add the yogurt, honey, lemon juice, and apples, and mix well.

Serve in bowls topped with 2 tablespoons of the blueberries per portion.

Serves 4

WLS portion ⅓ to ½

Calories per portion 290

Protein 8.1 g

Carbohydrate 57.6 g

Fat 3.4 g

Porridge with Apple, Cinnamon, and Pecans

Vegetarian

This superhealthy breakfast tastes like a delicious treat. The water-to-milk ratio can be adjusted according to your taste. The pecans are optional; simply omit them if you find you can't tolerate them at your post-op stage of eating.

- 1²/₃ cups old-fashioned rolled oats
- 1¾ cups low-fat milk, plus more as needed
- 1¼ cups water, plus more as needed
- ½ teaspoon ground cinnamon

- 2 dessert apples (such as Ginger Gold or Gala), peeled, cored, and grated (for a very soft texture) or finely chopped
- Sweetener, such as Splenda (optional)
- 6 pecans, chopped (optional)

Place the oats, milk, water, and cinnamon in a heavy-bottomed saucepan. Bring to a gentle simmer over medium-high heat, stirring frequently, and cook for 5 minutes or until thick and creamy. Add a splash more milk or water if the mixture is becoming too thick.

Stir in the apples. Add sweetener, if desired and tolerated.

Spoon into bowls and top with some of the pecans, if using. Serve immediately.

Serves 4
WLS portion ½
Calories per portion 230

Protein 10.1 g
Carbohydrate 37.8 g
Fat 4.6 g

Greek Yogurt with Honey, Berries, and Seeds

Vegetarian

This is a typical Greek dish showcasing some of the best ingredients of the country's cuisine: Greek yogurt, fragrant honey, and thyme. Mixed berries have been used here but you could just as easily use quartered ripe fresh figs. Omit the seeds if you have a problem with digesting them at an early stage and keep the honey to a minimum if you are very sugar sensitive. Serve this dish for breakfast, as an indulgent snack, or for dessert.

- 12 ounces fat-free Greek yogurt
- 12 ounces ripe mixed berries
- ¼ teaspoon fresh thyme leaves (optional)
- 2 tablespoons filtered Greek honey
- ¼ cup mixed seeds and nuts

Divide the yogurt among 4 plates and add an equal quantity of mixed berries on the side, tossed with the thyme leaves, if desired.

Drizzle the yogurt with a little of the honey and sprinkle a scattering of the mixed seeds and nuts on top.

Serve lightly chilled.

Serves 4

WLS portion ½

Calories per portion 155

Protein 6.6 g

Carbohydrate 20.2 g

Fat 4.9 g

Strawberry Soufflé Omelet

Vegetarian

This meltingly soft, wonderfully fluffy omelet rounds out a meal perfectly or makes a delicious and nutritious breakfast dish on a summer morning.

- 1½ cups sliced ripe strawberries
- 1 tablespoon lemon juice
- 3 tablespoons Splenda granulated sweetener
- 2 tablespoons water
- 4 large eggs, separated
- 1 teaspoon vanilla extract
- Low-fat butter-flavored cooking spray

Put the strawberries in a small pan with the lemon juice, half the sweetener, and the water. Heat gently until the fruit has softened slightly, about 2 minutes. Reduce the heat to very low.

Preheat the broiler to hot.

Beat the egg whites in a large bowl until stiff. In a separate bowl, beat the egg yolks with the remaining sweetener and the vanilla. Fold the egg yolk mixture into the egg whites with a large metal spoon.

Generously spritz a medium nonstick omelet pan or skillet with cooking spray. Heat over moderate heat until just hot. Add half the egg mixture and cook for about 1 minute, until the bottom of the omelet has just set. Place the pan under the broiler for a few moments until the top has set and browned a little.

Slice and transfer to a warmed serving plate, fill with half the strawberry mixture, and fold in half. Keep warm while you prepare the second omelet in the same way, then serve both immediately.

Serves 2

WLS portion ½ to ¾

Calories per portion 195

Protein 13.5 g

Carbohydrate 10.1 g

Fat 10.6 g

Creamy Lemon Blueberries

Vegetarian

Sometimes during the Soft Foods stage of eating, you yearn for something sweet yet zesty and indulgent. This dessert-like offering of tender blueberries layered with a tangy and creamy yogurt and cream cheese mixture fits the bill admirably—and all for less than 100 calories.

- 1 (7-ounce) container fat-free vanilla yogurt
- ½ cup fat-free cream cheese or other soft cheese
- 1 teaspoon honey
- 2 teaspoons finely grated lemon zest
- 2 cups fresh blueberries

Drain any excess liquid from the yogurt and place the yogurt in a bowl with the cream cheese and honey. Beat or whisk well until smooth and creamy. Fold in the lemon zest.

Layer the lemon mixture with the blueberries in four small dessert glasses. Cover and chill until ready to serve.

Serves 4

WLS portion ½ to 1

Calories per portion 100

Protein 7.4 g

Carbohydrate 15.3 g

Fat 0.2 g

Blueberry Compote Pudding

Vegetarian

This fruit-layered pudding is very simple to prepare and can be made well ahead and stored in the refrigerator. Make your own pudding or use ready-made pudding to save time.

- 2½ cups blueberries
- Splenda granulated sweetener
- Juice of ½ lemon
- 1 pound (about three 5-ounce containers) fat-free blueberry yogurt
- 1 cup prepared low-fat, low-sugar pudding
- ½ cup fat-free fromage blanc
- Zest of 1 lemon
- Fresh mint sprigs, for garnish

Set aside a few blueberries for decoration, then place the remainder in a small pan with a little sweetener (depending on the tartness of the berries) and the lemon juice. Bring to a boil, reduce the heat to maintain a simmer, and simmer for 3 to 4 minutes, until the berries begin to burst and release their juices. Remove from the heat and allow to cool completely.

In a bowl, combine the yogurt, pudding, fromage blanc, and lemon zest and mix well.

Spoon the cooked blueberry compote into the bottom of six serving glasses, then top with the pudding mixture. Chill for at least 3 hours before serving.

Serve decorated with the reserved blueberries and sprigs of fresh mint.

Serves 6

WLS portion ½

Calories per portion 107

Protein 5.9 g

Carbohydrate 19.5 g

Fat 0.8 g

Guilt-Free Chocolate Mousse

Vegan / Vegetarian

Here is an amazingly healthy alternative to conventional chocolate mousse. It's dairy-free, not too sweet, and cocoa-rich, but made buttery smooth with the addition of ripe avocado. It is sweetened with agave nectar rather than sugar or artificial sweetener (but can be made using the latter if preferred or to lower the calorie count—simply sweeten to taste as desired). Most bariatrics can tolerate agave nectar, but gastric bypass patients may want to stick to a smallish portion if unsure.

- 4 ripe avocados
- 1 cup agave nectar
- 1 tablespoon vanilla extract
- 1 cup unsweetened cocoa powder
- Fresh raspberries or other berries, for serving

Halve the avocados and remove the pits. Scoop the flesh into a food processor bowl and add the agave nectar, vanilla, and cocoa powder. Process until smooth, scraping down the sides of the bowl a few times during processing.

Alternatively, place the avocado flesh, agave nectar, vanilla, and cocoa powder in a bowl and beat with an electric whisk until smooth.

Spoon into small dessert dishes and chill thoroughly.

Serve chilled, topped with fresh berries.

Serves 8

WLS portion ½ to ¾

Calories per portion 233

Protein 3.8 g

Carbohydrate 25 g

Fat 15.9 g

Perfect Chocolate Truffles

Vegetarian

On special occasions like Christmas, Thanksgiving, Easter, and Valentine's Day, commercial chocolate offerings abound—but they do no favors for bariatrics, especially those susceptible to dumping syndrome (see page 11). So what's the alternative? These little low-fat and low-sugar morsels are perfect to end a meal or just offer a sweet treat when the call comes. If you prefer, substitute the drink powder with chocolate-flavored whey protein powder; use a generous scoop or 1½ ounces.

- 2 ounces dark chocolate
- 3 (½-ounce) packets low-fat, low-sugar chocolate drink powder
- 4 ounces low-fat cream cheese or other soft cheese
- 1½ teaspoons Splenda granulated sweetener

Break the chocolate pieces and place them in a bowl. Melt in the microwave or in a small heatproof bowl set over a pan of simmering water (do not let the bottom of the bowl touch the water).

Add 2 packets of the chocolate drink powder to the melted chocolate and mix well. Add the cream cheese and sweetener and mix well to form a smooth paste.

Chill for about 15 minutes or until firm enough to handle.

Pour the remaining packet of drink powder into a dish. Roll teaspoonfuls of the chilled chocolate mixture into small balls, then coat in the drink powder. Keep chilled until ready to serve.

Makes 16 truffles

WLS portion 1 to 2

Calories per truffle 29

Protein 1.3 g

Carbohydrate 3.4 g

Fat 1.1 g

Patriotic Cheesecake

Vegetarian / Suitable for Freezing

This delicious chilled cheesecake is called "patriotic" because it can be decorated with fresh berries to look like the American flag. It is made with orange sugar-free gelatin and ginger but can be adapted to make other flavor combinations by simply varying the flavor of gelatin and yogurt used. Good variations to try are Berry Delicious using raspberry geltain and strawberry yogurt; and Banoffee Dream using toffee yogurt with sliced bananas.

- 2 cups reduced-fat graham cracker crumbs
- 3 ounces low-fat spread or light butter, melted
- 1 teaspoon finely grated orange zest
- 2 (0.3 ounce) boxes (4-serving size) sugar-free orange gelatin crystals
- 1 cup boiling water
- 1¼ cups low-fat cream cheese or other soft cheese
- 7 ounces fat-free vanilla yogurt, stirred until smooth
- 1 ounce preserved young ginger in syrup, finely chopped
- Strawberries, raspberries, and blueberries, for garnish

Place the graham cracker crumbs in a bowl and add the melted low-fat spread and the orange zest. Mix well to coat, then spoon the crumb mixture into the base of a large serving dish or springform cake pan, pressing down firmly to make a base for the cheesecake. Transfer to the refrigerator to chill while you make the topping.

In a bowl, dissolve the gelatin crystals in the boiling water and allow to cool slightly.

Whisk the cream cheese and yogurt into the cooled gelatin mixture until smooth. Fold in the ginger. Pour the cheese mixture over the chilled crumb base, return to the refrigerator, and chill to firmly set, about 4 hours.

continued ▶

To serve, leave the cheesecake in the dish or unmold onto a plate. Decorate the top of the cheesecake with the berries to serve.

Serves 8   *Protein 8.9 g*

WLS portion ½ to ¾   *Carbohydrate 22.4 g*

Calories per portion 190   *Fat 7.1 g*

Banana and Prune Fool

Vegetarian

This literally takes just a couple of minutes to prepare yet is so tasty and seemingly indulgent. Thin to the desired consistency with the juice from the canned prunes.

- 5 canned prunes in unsweetened fruit juice, stones removed
- 1 small ripe banana, chopped
- 1 tablespoon fat-free Greek yogurt
- 1 tablespoon low-fat cream cheese or other soft cheese

Place all the ingredients in a small blender. Add 1 to 2 tablespoons of the juice from the canned prunes and puree until smooth.

Serve at once, or chill until ready to serve.

Serves 1

WLS portion ¾ to 1

Calories per portion 190

Protein 5.4 g

Carbohydrate 39.1 g

Fat 1.2 g

6

STAGE 5: EATING WELL FOR LIFE

Eating Well in Stage 5

Once you've grown accustomed to trying a variety of different foods during stages 3 and 4, you'll find that you're ready to move on to stage 5: Eating Well for Life. Most patients find that they reach this stage between eight and sixteen weeks after their operation—when they're able to eat a range of solid foods in small amounts.

Begin stage 5 with soft, moist foods. Serving food with some sauce, dressing, or gravy will make sure that every mouthful is moist and can travel through your new digestive system more easily. You should gradually cut down on these soft foods as you progress from week to week and go for more foods with a drier texture. These move more slowly through the body and will make you feel full for a longer period of time.

The Eating Well for Life stage is forever, so you shouldn't be in a rush to get there or to reach your goal weight—there's no race to the finish line. Remember to eat slowly, and learn to recognize when you're full so you don't eat beyond the feeling of satiety.

Gastric band patients, in particular, will learn to find their "sweet spot" during this time. This is when you're able to recognize you have eaten just the right amount—neither too much nor too little—so that you lose weight and feel comfortable and satisfied with it, and don't need too many adjustments to fill or de-fill your band.

If you cook and prepare meals for your partner or your family, now is the time (if you haven't already in the Soft Foods stage) to start making one meal for all of you to enjoy. Why waste time and money making different meals for yourself when the rest of the family will also benefit from your high-protein, low-fat, and low-sugar diet? You can always cook extra accompaniments for bigger appetites and an occasional sweet treat so that everyone gets a balanced, pleasurable diet.

Make good choices from all the recipes in this book and from a selection of advised foods in addition to taking a daily multivitamin, calcium supplement, and any other supplements prescribed or recommended by your bariatric team.

The Bariatric Mantra

High-protein, low-fat, and low-sugar is the mantra for bariatric eating. Here are the new rules and guidelines:

- Always eat your food in the right order. Protein comes first (meat, chicken, eggs, fish, and vegetable-based protein); vegetables and fruit come next; and then finally carbohydrates (pasta, rice, potatoes, and other starches).
- Protein should be as lean as possible. All visible fat, such as chicken skin or bacon rind, should be removed.
- Aim for a low-fat diet. Your food should ideally contain less than 5 g of fat per 100 g whenever possible.
- Choose low-sugar foods. Dumping syndrome (see page 11) can occur in gastric bypass patients if they eat more than 7 to 10 g sugar in one sitting. You'll soon know your limits.
- Eat three meals a day with a couple of small snacks in between if you are hungry.

- Beware of grazing, or eating small snacks throughout the day, as this will cause you to eat more than you realize.
- After the initial stages, opt for solid foods. Soft foods do slip down more easily but you often eat more of them without noticing.
- Slow down and chew every mouthful at least 20 times.
- Once you feel full, *stop eating.* Do not feel compelled to clear your plate.
- Keep your fluids up. Drink plenty throughout the day, but avoid drinking immediately before, during, or after a meal as it will fill up your new, much smaller stomach and encourage foods to pass more quickly through your digestive system.
- Get into the daily habit of taking a multivitamin, calcium supplement, and any other supplements your doctor recommends. This is imperative now that you can't eat nearly as much as you used to and will ensure your body gets all the nutrients it needs.
- Aim for 70 g of protein a day (or whatever amount your bariatric team recommends for you). This is a bit of a challenge and will be tough to start with, so consider using a whey protein isolate powder if you find you are struggling to eat the necessary levels. One protein powder drink can quickly provide you with an impressive 25 g of protein.

Warning Foods

There are quite a few warning foods that you may not tolerate well in the short or long term. Be aware of these and proceed with caution:
- Untoasted bread—especially soft and white varieties
- Overcooked pasta
- Mushy, overcooked rice
- Red meat with a fibrous texture like steak or chops
- Stringy vegetables like green beans

- Corn
- Pineapple
- Mushrooms with a tougher texture
- Pits, seeds, and skins from fruit and vegetables
- Dried fruit
- Popcorn
- Carbonated drinks and chewing gum—no caution here; these are banned for life.

Can Carbonated Drinks Really Blow Your Surgery?

One of the most popular questions from bariatric patients is "Do I really have to give up soda for good?"

Will a fizzy drink really jeopardize things? Sadly, the answer to this question is yes. Although some people find it tough to give up soda, there are some pretty compelling reasons why weight-loss surgery and carbonated drinks just don't mix.

The first is related to your new very small pouch or stomach size. Inflation of this can be uncomfortable and can cause stretching. For bypass and sleeve patients this can happen with just a mouthful—for gastric band patients, it can happen with only a sip.

Why does this happen? It's quite simple, really. As the gas comes out of the drink, it expands in your new small stomach just like a balloon, and if you keep repeatedly taking in the fizz, your stomach will stretch to a bigger size over time.

The second very good reason for kicking such drinks to the curb is because they have been shown to increase hunger (even the zero-calorie and low-sugar sodas), which means that you run the risk of regaining weight if you surrender to the hunger pangs.

So the general advice is that *any* drink that lists carbonated water as an ingredient—with or without added flavoring—is on the forbidden list.

What can you have instead? Well, it's obvious that water, tea, and coffee—hot or iced—are all okay, but you needn't restrict yourself to those alone. Why not consider zero-calorie and zero-fizz fruit-flavored waters and juices? Try fizz-free fruit-based "-ades" like orangeade and lemonade.

A cautionary note: Don't be tempted to guzzle sugary fruit juice instead. Its high sugar content may be problematic to gastric bypass patients and prove too caloric for others. The same can be said for some commercial fruit smoothies—so look for a bariatric smoothie recipe that can be made at home, where you're in control of the ingredients and the portion size. If you are going to drink fruit juice, make sure it's a reduced-sugar variety or 100% juice diluted with water.

Whatever you choose to supplement your water and fluid intake, remember the "no-drink rule" for band, bypass, and sleeve patients: Avoid drinking fluids for 30 minutes before and after a meal and while eating so that you don't flush food too quickly through your new stomach pouch.

Ten Tips for Low-Fat Cooking

Many recipes (including those aimed at dieters) contain high levels of undesirable nutrients, particularly saturated fat. Eating too much of this type of fat contributes to heart disease and obesity. For bariatric patients, following a low-fat diet is paramount to achieving weight-loss success and long-term maintenance.

Here are ten easy-to-follow rules that can make any recipe healthier by reducing the saturated fat content. Developed by the Fat Information Service, they are designed for anyone following a healthy-eating or weight-reducing diet. If you've been looking to adapt a presurgery favorite recipe for postsurgery eating, these simple tips to cut down or swap some ingredients could save the day.

1. If the recipe includes cream, replace it with low-fat fromage blanc, fat-free plain yogurt, or crème fraîche.

2. Swap whole milk for low-fat milk.

3. If you are choosing cheese to flavor a dish or sauce, opt for a strong-tasting one and use a smaller amount of it. Alternatively, try a reduced-fat version.

4. Swap butter for vegetable oil–based spreads or light butter.

5. Use unsaturated oils such as olive, sunflower, or grape seed instead of butter, lard, or ghee.

6. Wherever possible, broil meat, poultry, and fish instead of frying it, and cut off any visible fat or skin before cooking.

7. Use a nonstick pan to avoid adding extra fat when cooking, and consider spritzing the pan with nonstick cooking spray for sautéing.

8. Replace some of the meat in stews and casseroles with legumes and extra vegetables.

9. When making a pie, opt for just one crust—either a lid or a base. Also try making pastry with a vegetable oil–based spread instead of butter.

10. Broil, bake, poach, or steam foods instead of frying or roasting.

Smart Shopping Tips and Bargains for Smaller Appetites

Have you ever noticed how grocery shopping is aimed at getting us to buy extra food, thereby enticing us to eat more? Better deals on bigger quantities often make shopping more challenging for smaller households, or for those who just don't want or need to buy and cook more than is necessary.

So how can a weight-loss surgery patient or single diner manage this journey along the food aisles, downsize their shopping, and reduce their food waste on a budget? Here are a few ways:

- Have a plan. It sounds obvious, but it works. Creating a meal plan for the week or a few days at a time means you can shop sensibly. At the very least this prevents over-buying.

- Within that plan, go ahead and purchase certain items in larger quantities. But when you do buy big, buy wisely. Items like frozen fruit, vegetables, fish, and chicken pieces can be stored for months and dipped into when required. Likewise, dried items like pasta, rice, legumes, and some cereals can be good investments—just ensure their packaging can be resealed to preserve quality.

- Take advantage of coupons for those items you buy regularly, but beware of those that just tempt you to overindulge. If temptation does get the better of you, at least try to make sure it's an item that stores well.

- Stock up on individually portioned or single-serving packages. It's true that we all want to cut back on packaging, but this may be the one time you will benefit from a little more. The physical barrier of having to open a second portioned packet of cookies, crackers, or nuts might help you scale back and prevent overeating. It will also cut back on food waste.

- Many items on supermarket shelves are geared to larger house-holds, so a bunch of bananas might have 8, a stem of tomatoes might hold 6, and a bunch of grapes might satisfy a family of 6. Feel obliged to take only what you need: divide the bananas, pull off a couple of tomatoes from their stem, and halve or quarter the bunch of grapes. Obviously this is for fruit and vegetables sold by weight, not by package, but you get the idea.

- Shop the salad bar for salad or chopped fruit and vegetables, taking just what you need for a salad, stir-fry, or main meal recipe. No need to leave the excess quantity of such items to linger in the crisper drawer for days until they wilt and perish, then need to be thrown in the trash.

- Likewise, shop the meat, fish, bakery, and deli counters rather than the food aisles. Ask for a single portion for a hamburger, fish dish, or lunchtime meal, or request that larger quantities be divided and then wrapped individually for the freezer.
- Cook items like rice, beans, and grains well ahead and freeze them. Use the whole, larger, better-value package, then remove what you require for the immediate meal and freeze the remainder. These items store well for up to 3 months and will save you time (and fuel) when cooking your next rice-, bean-, or grain-based meal.
- Scan the discounted foods shelves. Many smaller items find their way to this shelf and won't suit those buying for a family. A single small steak filet, a tiny salmon fillet, or a few slices of cooked meat might mean that you score a big bargain or two.
- Finally, cook from scratch. That way you know what you're eating, you can tailor quantities for one or two servings, and you won't waste the excess food on a meal designed for four people or more. Most recipes can be scaled down to one or two portions.

Dining Out, Bariatric Gourmet–Style

Restaurant stress is a very real worry for those both pre- and post-op. "Will I be able to dine out?" "What will I be able to eat?" "What if there is nothing I feel I can eat on the menu?" "What about drinks?"

These are all valid questions, but they shouldn't hamper your social dining if you follow these tips:

- Prepare ahead and check out the menu at the restaurant. Most restaurants have a website to browse or a menu posted out front, and many that don't will e-mail or fax a copy if you ask them. Then you can decide ahead of time what you want to order before you arrive. It will also give you the chance to plan any substitutions that you might want to ask for.

- Ask for substitutions. Don't be afraid to do this.
- Most restaurants are happy to serve you two starters instead of a starter and a main dish.
- Hold the dressing or sauce, or ask for it on the side.
- Ask for the dish to be prepared without added oil or butter, or with minimal amounts.
- Flash a weight-loss surgery request card, if you wish. Some charities and support groups have produced their own, which can be discreetly shown to the waitstaff or manager. Such cards request that you be allowed to be served a child-size portion.
- If you're concerned about portion size, why not consider sharing a plate with your fellow diners? Sharing plates is very popular on menus at the moment, and no one blinks an eye at anyone requesting a dessert with two spoons.
- It's often easier to take the glass of water and leave it untouched rather than refuse it and feel the need to explain why. Keeping it full and in front of you also means the waitstaff won't feel the need to keep topping it off; just don't drink it. Wondering if you will be tempted to have just a sip or two? Dose it heavily with salt—that quickly kills the desire.
- Ask for a doggie bag for leftover food. If you're sure you won't eat all the food you ordered, or know that the portion sizes are large where you are dining, ask for half of the food to be bagged before it is served.
- Don't draw attention to yourself—most people only care about what is on their plate rather than on yours. Take your time with your meal, pace yourself with your companions, and *enjoy* your own few mouthfuls.

All dining establishments want you to be happy with your order and want you to come back again. You don't have to tell them you've had weight-loss surgery—to them, you're just a customer.

To Booze or Not to Booze: That Is the Question

And a very controversial question it is. In all seriousness, this is one to discuss with your bariatric team, and then be sure to follow their advice.

Some surgeons give an emphatic *no*—others say yes, but with a cautionary note. Almost all, without exception, will advise bariatric patients never to have alcohol within the first 6 to 12 months post-op.

The reason? Your liver will be working hard to deal with all the weight-loss products your body is producing while losing weight quickly, so it doesn't need to contend with the additional workload of alcohol breakdown.

After the first 6 to 12 months, some alcohol may be tolerated, but with extreme care. One thing is for sure—your new bariatric replumbing and setup will probably mean that you can't tolerate alcohol the way you might have been able to prior to surgery.

In short, you become the "cheap date"—just one glass may make you feel intoxicated in no time at all. It's as if the alcohol is fast-tracked into your bloodstream with the speed of an F1 race car.

For this reason, it makes sense to never drink alone (keep yourself safe with responsible family and friends) unless you know your tolerance levels very well. Never, ever drink and drive, even after just one drink. Measured levels of alcohol in the bloodstream and in the body of individuals post-op have been proven to be higher than those of non–weight-loss surgery drinkers who imbibed the same amounts. You would probably fail a breath test, and your ability to judge distances and so on would be impaired.

With regard to weight, it's better to avoid sugary and high-fat or creamy alcoholic drinks for the calories alone, but gastric bypass patients may also find them unwelcome triggers for dumping syndrome (see page 11).

On a practical level, avoid carbonated alcoholic beverages—if a drink offered is slightly sparkling, then swirl it with a spoon or swizzle stick to get rid of as much gas as possible as a last resort. Ice cubes will do a similar job.

Better still is to check out some nonalcoholic options. Consider heavily diluted fruit juices, flavored waters (with no added sugar), sugar-free cordials and syrups made with ice water, iced tea, coffee drinks with artificial sweeteners, or alcohol-free wine. The latter now comes in red, white and rosé; there's even a lightly sparkling white that makes a fabulous replacement for champagne; just stir it well to reduce the bubbles before drinking so they won't inflate your stomach pouch.

Setting Up a Support System

It can be a tough call to stay motivated when it comes to sustained weight loss, maintenance, and fitness goals. Many coaches recommend that one of the best ways is to have a solid network of friends, family, and other supporters to help you accomplish your goals. But what if your family lives miles away, friends aren't available 24–7, or your loved ones aren't as enthusiastic or supportive as you'd like them to be?

Well, with a little know-how, you can overcome these obstacles and put your own cheerleading support system in place for when the going gets tough. Here are a few ways to stay motivated on your own:

- Find some virtual friends. Forums, message boards, and other online communities enable you to make friends with like-minded people regardless of where you—or they—live. Log on, listen, and if you feel like it, have a chat.
- Set a little challenge for yourself. Aim for something doable and achievable, but that needs just a little extra push. Perhaps one of your virtual buddies can join you in the challenge.
- Commit to a weekly weigh-in (but not more often). Even if it's just with a log-on weight-monitoring setup, it serves as a reminder of how far you have come. Or check in with a supportive family

member or a friend once a week with a weigh-in update. It might be just what you need to help stay on track.

- Set up a reward system for yourself. Throw a dollar or two in a jar for every pound you lose or every exercise session completed, then use it later for a healthy treat.
- Give yourself a pep talk to reaffirm your goals from time to time; write a regular journal that sets out your goals, struggles, setbacks, successes, and accomplishments; or take some photos or make a video diary that reminds you of your journey. It can be a great way to support yourself when there is no one else around to do so.
- Supporters don't just have to be people. Enlist your pet as your workout partner. Think of your dog or horse, for example, as your daily motivator: They always need, and rarely decline, an exercise opportunity.
- Finally, surround yourself with success. Indulge yourself with feel-good stories of those who have succeeded. Many are featured in magazines, in books, and on TV, including on weight-loss reality shows. Such stories can lift your spirits when your motivation is flagging, and reading or watching how someone else has pushed through their limitations may be all you need to help you through some tricky times, too.

How to Say "No, Thank You"

Pre-op, it's often hard to eat healthy, calorie-controlled food when there's so much food available, and it's especially difficult post-op when you can only eat small portions from a restricted range. However, one of the most challenging scenarios is when well-meaning family members, friends, and coworkers offer you food and you need to decline. How can you do this in a gracious way?

- It's always best to start with a simple and direct "No, thank you." Job done? Sadly, sometimes not, so here are some more ways to respond to those persistent "food pushers":
- Thanks, but I've already eaten.
- Looks fabulous—too good to eat!
- Thanks, I'll have some later.
- I'm good, thanks.
- Thank you, but I'm trying to eat healthier.
- I have a weigh-in tomorrow, so I'm reining in tonight and on my best behavior.
- No, thanks, but I'd love the recipe!
- What a shame I'm allergic to _____ [ingredient in the dish].
- I don't have any room on my plate at the moment. I'll try some later.
- I'm just too full at the moment.
- I'm saving my calories for _____ [insert another dish that you know might be coming up].
- I need a break from food right now—I've been cooking all day!
- No thanks, but I know my husband/wife/partner/friend is just dying to try it!
- I'm just a whisker away from my goal weight, so I'm going to say no today.
- I ate some when I arrived, and it's great.

And for those drink pushers:

- I'm the designated driver tonight [or volunteer if required].
- I can't drink with my medication.
- I have some tests scheduled tomorrow, so I'll have to refuse.

Six Ways to Celebrate Your Weight Loss Without Food

When we think of celebrating, many of us rejoice with food or a special edible treat. However, when celebrating weight loss, especially after bariatric surgery, food is not the best thing to choose.

Restriction in terms of portion size and food choice can limit your options considerably, so why not look at other ways to celebrate the pounds you have lost or a special milestone you have achieved along the way?

- Check out a new hobby and splurge on the "ingredients" needed. For example, try making your own jewelry; knitting or embroidering some unique design; or molding a piece of pottery. Make it eventful by adding a special charm to your jewelry to mark a specific loss or target; incorporate a pertinent message into your knitted or sewn design; or inscribe your pottery with your name and the date of your "surgi-versary" or when you reached your target weight.
- Celebrate by doing something daring that you couldn't have done before due to the limitations of excess weight. Think about skydiving, bungee jumping, rappelling, or doing an endurance challenge. Make it all the sweeter by getting sponsors and giving the proceeds to your favorite charity.
- Compare your weight loss to other things. Do an Internet search for things that weigh approximately the amount you have lost. You might have lost the weight of a kangaroo, 50 packs of butter, 15 typical newborn babies, or 2 supermodels!
- Have a special photograph taken. After hiding away behind the camera for years, you deserve it. Splurge by getting it taken by a professional (and bring in experts to help with makeup, hair, and clothes). Then frame it and display it for all to see.
- Save the money you would normally spend on food treats and use it to invest in a piece of health equipment or a gym membership.

A new bike, treadmill, pair of quality walking shoes, or one-day spa treat would be great options. Or buy yourself a new cookbook, health manual, or motivational guide.

- Book that once-in-a-lifetime or never-in-your-previous-lifetime vacation. This might be a long haul on a flight where you can now comfortably buckle that airline seat belt (without an extension) and pull down the food tray to knee level; a second honeymoon to somewhere you have always dreamed of; or just a day trip to a theme park where previously you couldn't enjoy the rides. Life now has many more options.

Breakfast and Lunch Ideas

Breakfast Ideas for Stage 5

- Any of the breakfast options suitable for stages 1, 2, 3, and 4 (see pages 18, 29, 55, and 90)
- Whole-wheat toast with low-fat spread or light butter and sugar-free jam, pure fruit puree, or smooth peanut butter
- Any "no-added-sugar" breakfast cereal with low-fat milk
- Porridge with fruit, such as strawberries or blueberries
- Shredded Wheat with dried fruit and low-fat milk
- Fresh fruit salad with low-fat fromage blanc
- Poached egg and whole-wheat toast
- Two-egg omelet with mushrooms or other vegetables or low-fat cream cheese or other soft cheese
- Small portion of low-sugar baked beans with whole-wheat toast
- Grapefruit segments, a baked egg, and whole-wheat toast
- Low-fat and low-sugar cereal bar
- Homemade low-fat and low-sugar breakfast muffin
- Low-fat and low-sugar muesli or granola with low-fat milk
- Vegetable and low-fat cheese frittata
- Cottage cheese or low-fat ricotta cheese pancakes
- Baked French toast made with whole-wheat bread

Lunches for Stage 5

- Any of the options listed for stages 1, 2, 3, and 4 (see pages 18, 29, 55, and 90)
- Baked potato with a topping, such as tuna, baked beans, or grated low-fat or cottage cheese
- Wedge of frittata or Spanish omelet with a little salad
- Portion of crustless quiche with a little salad

- Small portion of stir-fried vegetables with meat, fish, or meat alternative
- Whole-wheat pasta with a tomato-based sauce
- Grilled fish fingers with a little mashed potato and some peas
- Brown rice or whole-wheat pasta salad with chopped meat or flaked fish, tomatoes, and low-fat mayonnaise
- Mackerel or sardines on toast
- Whole-wheat bread sandwich, pita, or wrap with meat, fish, cheese, egg, or mixed vegetables and salad
- Low-fat sausage and grilled tomatoes and mushrooms
- Meat, fish, or vegetable kebabs with a little brown rice
- Small salad with meat, fish, eggs, beans, or low-fat cheese

Eating Well for Life Stage Recipes

- Aromatic Chicken with Chickpeas (page 152)
- Mediterranean Chicken Burgers (page 154)
- Creamy Curried Chicken with Apricots (page 156)
- Chicken with Pesto and Parma Ham (page 157)
- Yakitori Kebabs (page 158)
- One-Pan Sesame Lemon Chicken (page 159)
- Chicken and Basil Pizza (page 161)
- Turkey and Lemon Stir-Fry (page 162)
- Roast Turkey with Couscous and Apricot Stuffing (page 163)
- Lamb Koftas with Yogurt and Mint Dip (page 166)
- Pork and Apple Meatballs (page 168)
- Oven-Baked Ham (page 170)
- Crustless Quiche with Ham (page 171)
- Sweet Potato, Broccolini, and Bacon Hash (page 173)
- Pasta-Free Lasagna (page 174)
- Steak with Pepper Salsa (page 176)
- Pollock and Shrimp Biryani (page 177)

- Cod on a Pepper Bed (page 179)
- Salmon with Chunky Ratatouille (page 180)
- Wild Alaskan Salmon Celebration Roast (page 182)
- Thai Steamed Salmon (page 183)
- Tuna Steaks with Mango-Avocado Salad (page 184)
- Warm Leek, Smoked Trout, and Potato Salad (page 185)
- Salade Niçoise (page 186)
- Italian Bean and Sardine Salad (page 188)
- Greek Salad (page 190)
- Warm Green Bean, Halloumi, and Potato Salad (page 191)
- Warm Goat Cheese with Pear and Pecan Salad (page 193)
- Chickpea and Broccoli Frittata (page 195)
- Pumpkin, Bean, and Tomato Risotto (page 197)
- Israeli Couscous with Roasted Vegetables (page 199)
- Nutty Amaretti-Stuffed Peaches (page 201)
- Apple and Pineapple Kebabs with Ginger-Yogurt Dip (page 202)
- Apple Berry Crumble (page 203)
- Pear-Ginger Cake (page 204)
    Variation: Apple-Cinnamon Cake (page 205)
- Banana-Walnut Tea Bread (page 206)
- Pumpkin Bread (page 207)
- Cream Cheese–Frosted Cupcakes (page 209)
- Celebratory Carrot Cake (page 211)

Aromatic Chicken with Chickpeas

Suitable for Freezing

This gently spiced chicken dish is ideal for a simple weekday family meal, and with all the ingredients in the same pot, it's easy to clean up, too. Ras el hanout is a Moroccan spice blend with the wonderful warming flavor tones of many spices like cardamom, cinnamon, paprika, chili, and turmeric, and is well worth seeking out from international food stores and suppliers. If you have a problem with spicy food, the spice blend can be omitted from the recipe with perfectly good results. This dish is very good served with couscous.

- Low-fat nonstick cooking spray
- 1 onion, chopped
- 2 carrots, halved lengthwise and sliced into half-moons
- 11 ounces skinless and boneless chicken breast, cut into strips
- 1 tablespoon *ras el hanout* spice mix
- 1 (14-ounce) can chopped tomatoes
- 1¼ cups hot chicken stock
- 1 (14-ounce) can chickpeas, drained and rinsed
- Salt and freshly ground black pepper
- 3 to 4 tablespoons chopped cilantro leaves(optional)

Spritz a large, heavy-bottomed saucepan generously with cooking spray. Heat over low heat, add the onion and carrots, cover, and cook for about 10 minutes.

Remove the vegetables from the pan with a slotted spoon and set aside. Raise the heat slightly, add the chicken strips, and cook until golden on all sides.

Stir in the *ras el hanout* and cook for 1 minute. Return the vegetables to the pan and add the tomatoes and stock. Stir in the chickpeas and salt and pepper to taste. Bring to a simmer, cover, and cook, stirring occasionally, for 20 minutes or until the chicken is tender.

Stir in the cilantro, if using, and serve.

Serves 4
WLS portion ½
Calories per portion 225

Protein 30.3 g
Carbohydrate 16.9 g
Fat 4.1 g

Mediterranean Chicken Burgers

Forget the fast-food burger in a bun dripping with cheese and sauce—and fat and calories. Here's a fresh and light burger with an inspired herby twist, topped with tomato relish. If you really do yearn for some cheese with your burger, why not bury a small disc of extra-light cheese (like Babybel) in the center of the burger before broiling? It oozes out beautifully when you bite into the burger.

For the burgers

- 1 pound ground chicken (or the ground meat from about 4 skinless and boneless chicken breasts)
- 1 garlic clove, crushed
- Zest of 1 lemon
- 2 teaspoons sun-dried tomato paste
- 1 teaspoon chopped fresh basil leaves
- 1 egg white, lightly beaten
- Salt and freshly ground black pepper
- Low-fat nonstick cooking spray

For the relish

- ¼ cup chopped fresh flat-leaf parsley leaves
- 1 tablespoon chopped fresh basil leaves
- 1 shallot, finely chopped
- 2 tomatoes, peeled, seeded, and finely chopped
- Juice of 1 lemon
- Salt and freshly ground black pepper

To prepare the burgers: In a large bowl, combine the chicken, garlic, lemon zest, sun-dried tomato paste, basil, egg white, and salt and pepper to taste, mixing well. Divide the mixture into 8 equal portions and form them into patties.

Preheat the broiler to medium.

Place a sheet of foil on a broiler rack and spritz generously with cooking spray. Place the burgers on the foil and spray lightly with cooking spray. Broil for 5 to 6 minutes on each side.

Meanwhile, to prepare the relish: In a small bowl, combine the parsley, basil, shallot, tomatoes, lemon juice, and salt and pepper to taste.

Serve the cooked burgers with the relish.

Serves 4

WLS portion ½ (1 burger)

Calories per portion 167

Protein 27.9 g

Carbohydrate 4.1 g

Fat 3.6 g

Creamy Curried Chicken with Apricots

This very tasty cold dish of cooked chicken mixed with a lightly curried mayonnaise and pieces of fresh mango and dried apricot is fabulous to serve as part of a buffet with other salads. Vegetarians can use a meat substitute (like cooked Quorn chicken-style pieces) instead of the chicken.

- ⅓ cup fat-free mayonnaise
- ⅓ cup fat-free plain yogurt or orange yogurt
- 2 teaspoons medium curry paste (such as for tikka masala)
- Zest and juice of 1 orange
- 1 teaspoon grated peeled fresh ginger
- 1 teaspoon finely chopped red chili (optional)
- 2 teaspoons mango chutney
- 4 cooked skinless and boneless chicken breasts, cut into bite-size pieces
- 1 red onion, finely chopped
- 4 soft dried apricots, chopped
- 1 mango, pitted, peeled, and chopped
- Salt and freshly ground black pepper
- 1 tablespoon toasted sliced almonds
- Arugula leaves, for garnish

In a medium bowl, combine the mayonnaise, yogurt, curry paste, orange zest and juice, ginger, chili (if using), and mango chutney and mix well to make a smooth sauce.

Add the chicken, onion, apricots, chopped mango, and salt and pepper to taste, mixing well.

Spoon into a serving dish, scatter the almonds on top, and serve garnished with a few arugula leaves.

Serves 4

WLS portion ½

Calories per portion 275

Protein 31.8 g

Carbohydrate 22.1 g

Fat 6.9 g

Chicken with Pesto and Parma Ham

Here is a fantastic chicken entrée that is easy to make, looks impressive, and is loaded with protein. You could use red pesto or sun-dried tomato paste instead of the traditional green pesto, if preferred.

- 4 (4-ounce) skinless and boneless chicken breasts
- 4 teaspoons pesto
- 3 ounces thinly sliced Parma ham
- 12 fresh basil leaves
- 1 pound baby carrots, halved

- 2 bell peppers, cored, seeded, and cut into chunks
- 1 large red onion, sliced into thin wedges
- Salt and freshly ground black pepper
- Low-fat nonstick cooking spray

Preheat oven to 375°F.

Using a sharp knife, slice a pocket into each chicken breast, being careful not to cut all the way through, and open it up. Spread 1 teaspoon of the pesto into each breast, then divide the Parma ham slices evenly among them. Top with the basil leaves, then close the pockets and secure them with wooden toothpicks or small skewers.

Place the carrots, bell peppers, red onion, and salt and black pepper to taste in a roasting pan and spritz generously with cooking spray. Arrange the chicken breasts on top.

Cook in the oven for 25 to 30 minutes, or until the chicken is cooked through and the vegetables are tender. Serve immediately.

Serves 4

WLS portion ½

Calories per portion 275

Protein 33 g

Carbohydrate 20.4 g

Fat 7.2 g

Yakitori Kebabs

Yakitori is Japanese for marinated chicken kebabs. This recipe also has marinated Romano peppers in the mix. You can, of course, use bell peppers or pieces of zucchini instead. If you are short on time, marinate the chicken for just 20 minutes—it will still absorb a lot of the flavors. Serve with rice noodles, if desired and tolerated.

- Generous ¼ cup soy sauce
- 3 tablespoons mirin
- 1 tablespoon filtered honey
- 1 tablespoon grated peeled fresh ginger
- 1 garlic clove, crushed

- 1 pound skinless and boneless chicken breast, cubed
- 4 scallions, cut into thirds
- 1 Romano pepper, cored, seeded, and cut into chunks
- Rice noodles, for serving (optional)

In a large bowl, mix the soy sauce with the mirin, honey, ginger, and garlic. Add the chicken and stir well. Cover and leave to marinate in the refrigerator for at least 1 to 2 hours or overnight.

Preheat the broiler to medium-high. Thread the chicken, scallions, and Romano pepper onto four metal skewers, alternating the ingredients as you go; reserve the marinade.

Place the kebabs on the broiler rack and brush them liberally with the reserved marinade. Broil for 10 to 15 minutes, turning occasionally and basting with the marinade. The chicken should be cooked until the juices run clear, and the vegetables are slightly charred.

Serve immediately with rice noodles, if desired and tolerated.

Serves 4

WLS portion ½

Calories per portion (without noodles) 200

Protein 30 g

Carbohydrate 13.5 g

Fat 2.7 g

One-Pan Sesame Lemon Chicken

This is a super-relaxed chicken dish that has everything in one pan. It's good for entertaining family and friends and can easily be doubled up to serve more. Cooked rice makes a good accompaniment.

- 8 skinless and boneless chicken thigh fillets
- 1 large butternut squash (about 2¼ pounds), peeled, seeded, and cut into bite-size chunks
- 1 head garlic, broken into cloves, unpeeled
- Salt and freshly ground black pepper
- Low-fat nonstick cooking spray
- 2 lemons, quartered
- 8 ounces broccolini
- 2 tablespoons filtered honey
- 2 tablespoons sesame seeds
- Cooked rice, for serving (optional)

Preheat oven to 350°F.

Lay the chicken in a large roasting pan and scatter the butternut squash pieces and garlic cloves around it. Season with salt and pepper and generously spritz with cooking spray. Squeeze the juice from the lemon quarters over the chicken and tuck the squeezed lemon peels in and around the chicken and squash.

Bake for 40 minutes, until the chicken is just about cooked through and the squash is soft.

Meanwhile, bring a saucepan of water to a boil. Blanch the broccolini for 2 minutes, drain, and set aside.

Remove the pan from the oven and stir in the blanched broccolini, coating it well in the lemony juices. Drizzle the honey all over and sprinkle with the sesame seeds.

continued ▶

Return the pan to the oven for 10 minutes more, until the chicken is sticky and golden. Serve at once, with rice, if desired and tolerated.

Serves 4

WLS portion ½

Calories per portion (without rice) 420

Protein 37.5 g

Carbohydrate 25.4 g

Fat 18.7 g

Chicken and Basil Pizza

Never thought you could have pizza again after weight-loss surgery? Well, you can. Okay, so it's not the fat-laden, deep-dish, stuffed-crust kind anymore, but there is a lighter and healthier version. Here it is topped with chicken, basil, and cheese, but you could try countless other variations with tuna, egg, shrimp, deli meats, and vegetables.

- 1 low-carb or whole-wheat tortilla
- 2 tablespoons tomato salsa (store-bought, or see page 69)
- ¼ cup chopped cooked boneless and skinless chicken breast
- 6 cherry tomatoes, halved
- 1 (4-ounce) ball low-fat or part-skim mozzarella, thinly sliced
- 6 anchovy fillets
- 1 tablespoon grated Parmesan
- Salt and freshly ground black pepper
- Fresh basil leaves, for garnish

Preheat oven to 375°F.

Lightly grease a baking sheet or line it with a nonstick reusable baking liner. Place the tortilla on top.

Spread the tomato salsa evenly over the tortilla. Top with the chicken, cherry tomatoes, mozzarella, anchovies, Parmesan, and salt and pepper to taste.

Bake for 10 to 12 minutes. Cut into wedges and serve, garnished with fresh basil.

Serves 2

WLS portion ½

Calories per portion 245

Protein 22 g

Fat 12.3 g

Turkey and Lemon Stir-Fry

Here is an everyday low-fat stir-fry recipe using turkey breast fillets; you could use chicken just as well. The crunchy stir-fry vegetable ingredients are up to you—what do you have left in your crisper drawer? Here, there's broccoli, carrots, and a little red cabbage and onion, but you can use almost anything or your favorite combination. It's the lemon and ginger that allow this ordinary dish to become something truly special.

- 8 ounces skinless and boneless turkey breast
- 1 teaspoon Chinese five-spice powder
- Low-fat nonstick cooking spray
- 5 ounces prepared stir-fry vegetables (onion, broccoli, carrots and red cabbage, for example)
- Zest and juice of 1 lemon
- 1 teaspoon grated peeled fresh ginger
- 2 tablespoons soy sauce
- Salt and freshly ground black pepper
- Cooked noodles or rice, for serving (optional)

Cut the turkey into thin slices and toss it with the five-spice powder to coat.

Generously spritz a wok or nonstick skillet with cooking spray and heat over medium-high heat until hot. Add the turkey and stir-fry for 3 to 4 minutes until just cooked through. Remove and set aside.

Spritz the pan again with cooking spray, add the vegetable mixture, and stir-fry for 3 minutes or until almost tender.

Return the turkey to the pan and add the lemon zest, lemon juice, ginger, soy sauce, and salt and pepper to taste, mixing well. Cook for 1 minute more.

Serve with noodles or rice, if desired and tolerated.

Serves 2

WLS portion ½

Calories per portion (without noodles or rice) 168

Protein 33 g

Carbohydrate 5.4 g

Fat 1.4 g

Roast Turkey with Couscous and Apricot Stuffing

Vegan / Vegetarian

Here's the Thanksgiving, Christmas, or celebration turkey you have been waiting for. It's a holiday favorite that is lighter than the original presurgery choice. The stuffing here is made from couscous flavored with onion, herbs, and nuts and can be cooked inside the turkey or outside (your choice). Serve with homemade cranberry sauce (see the tip at the end of this recipe).

For the stuffing

- Scant 1 cup dried couscous
- 2 garlic cloves, crushed
- 1 small onion, finely chopped
- 5 ounces zucchini, coarsely grated
- 1 tablespoon chopped fresh sage
- 2 ounces soft dried apricots, finely chopped
- ¼ cup sliced almonds, toasted
- Salt and freshly ground black pepper
- 6 thin bacon slices, halved (optional)

For the turkey

- One 12-pound turkey
- 2 oranges, cut into wedges
- 1¼ cups dry white wine
- 2 tablespoons cornstarch
- Bay leaves, for garnish

To prepare the stuffing: Put the couscous in a bowl and add enough boiling water to cover the couscous by about ½ inch. Cover the bowl and let stand for 10 minutes, then fluff with a fork to separate the grains. Add the garlic, onion, zucchini, sage, apricots, almonds, and salt and pepper to taste, mixing well. Allow to cool.

Preheat oven to 375°F.

Use the stuffing to stuff the neck cavity of the turkey. Alternatively, spoon it into small molds or ramekins, each lined with half a slice of

continued ▶

bacon, if desired. These can then be cooked for the last 20 to 30 minutes of the cooking time, alongside the turkey, or while the turkey is resting.

To prepare the turkey: Place the orange wedges inside the body cavity of the turkey, then carefully place the turkey in a roasting pan (do not dislodge the couscous stuffing if you have used it to stuff the neck cavity). Pour the wine into the pan and cover the turkey tightly with foil. Roast for 3½ hours, removing the foil for the final 20 to 30 minutes of cooking (this is a good time to place the individual portions of stuffing in the oven if you have not placed the stuffing in the turkey) or until the turkey is cooked. To check, pierce the thickest part of the thigh with a skewer—if the turkey is done, the juices that run out should be clear with no traces of pink. Transfer to a carving plate, re-cover with foil, and leave in a warm place to rest for up to 1 hour before serving.

To make the gravy, pour off the juices from the roasting pan into a measuring cup or gravy separator and set aside to allow them to settle. When settled, skim off any visible fat (the clear or yellowish top layer). You should have about 2½ cups of juices; if there isn't quite enough, top off the measuring cup with hot turkey or vegetable stock. Mix the cornstarch with a little water. Heat the turkey juices in a small saucepan. Whisk in the cornstarch mixture and cook, stirring constantly, until the gravy is smooth and thickened.

Serve the turkey with the stuffing and gravy, garnished with bay leaves.

Serves 6   *Protein 28.8 g*
WLS portion ½   *Carbohydrate 25.5 g*
Calories per portion 295   *Fat 8.4 g*

TIP
Cranberry Sauce

Roast turkey is delicious with cranberry sauce. Make your own low-sugar variation with this recipe.

- Two 8-ounce packages fresh or frozen whole cranberries
- Zest and juice of 1 small orange
- ½ cup Splenda granulated sweetener
- 1 cinnamon stick

Pick over the cranberries then rinse them well. Place in a saucepan with the orange zest and juice, sweetener, and cinnamon. Bring to a boil, then reduce the heat to maintain a simmer. Simmer, stirring occasionally, for 15 to 20 minutes, until the berries have burst and produced a thick sauce.

Allow to cool slightly before serving, or let cool then refrigerate until needed. Remove and discard the cinnamon stick before serving.

Serves 6

WLS portion ¼ to ½

Calories per portion 28

Protein 0.5 g

Carbohydrate 6.9 g

Fat 0.1 g

Lamb Koftas with Yogurt and Mint Dip

These cheese and lamb meatballs can be cooked on the grill or broiled, depending on the weather. You also don't have to be a purist with the meat; if you prefer, simply substitute lean ground beef, turkey, or chicken for the lamb. It is important, however, to use a good strong cheddar for the recipe. A mature, strong-tasting cheese means that you don't have to use too much to get a fine flavor. Serve with salad and pita bread, if you can tolerate it.

For the koftas

- 1 pound lean ground lamb
- ¾ cup finely grated aged sharp cheddar
- 1 teaspoon ground allspice
- 1 small onion, very finely chopped
- 1 garlic clove, crushed

- 1 teaspoon finely grated lemon zest
- 2 teaspoons dried mixed herbs, or 4 teaspoons chopped fresh mixed herbs
- Salt and freshly ground black pepper

For the dip

- 1 (5-ounce) container fat-free Greek yogurt
- ½ cup low-fat hummus (see page 66)

- 2 teaspoons chopped fresh mint leaves
- Salt and freshly ground black pepper

To serve

- Salad (optional)

- Pita bread (optional)

Soak eight wooden skewers in warm water while you prepare the meat mixture (this prevents them from scorching during cooking).

To prepare the koftas: Preheat the broiler or start the coals in an outdoor grill.

In a large bowl, mix the lamb with the cheese, allspice, onion, garlic, lemon zest, herbs, and salt and pepper to taste. Form the mixture into balls, then thread them onto the soaked skewers.

Cook under the broiler or over medium coals on the grill for 8 to 10 minutes, turning frequently.

Meanwhile, to prepare the dip: In a small bowl, combine the yogurt, hummus, mint, and salt and pepper.

Serve the cooked koftas with the dip and salad and pita bread, if desired.

Serves 4

WLS portion ½

Calories per portion (without salad or pita) 370

Protein 30.9 g

Carbohydrate 10.8 g

Fat 22.5 g

Pork and Apple Meatballs

Suitable for Freezing

Meatballs made with ground pork and grated apple, simmered in a simple tomato sauce, make a lovely midweek meal that will be popular with bariatrics and their families alike. Change the sauce by choosing a passata or crushed tomato mixture with peppers or chilies instead of the onion and garlic for variety. All taste great with a serving of freshly cooked pasta, if you can tolerate it, or zucchini "pasta" ribbons.

- 1 pound cooking apples (such as Northern Spy or Pink Lady), peeled, quartered, and cored
- 1 pound extra-lean ground pork
- 1½ cups soft fresh whole-wheat bread crumbs
- 2 teaspoons dried sage, or 1 teaspoon chopped fresh sage leaves
- 1 egg yolk, beaten
- Salt and freshly ground black pepper
- Low-fat nonstick cooking spray
- 1 (24-ounce) jar passata or crushed tomatoes with onion and garlic
- Cooked pasta, for serving (optional)

Coarsely grate the apples and place half in a large bowl. Add the ground pork, bread crumbs, sage, egg yolk, and salt and pepper to taste. Bind the mixture together with your hands then divide and shape it into about 32 small meatballs.

Generously spritz a large nonstick skillet with cooking spray. Heat over high heat, then add the meatballs in batches and fry, stirring and turning occasionally, for 6 to 8 minutes until golden brown on all sides.

Add the remaining apple and stir well. Add the passata and salt and pepper to taste. Cover and simmer for 5 to 7 minutes or until the sauce has thickened slightly.

Serve hot, over freshly cooked pasta, if desired.

Serves 4

WLS portion ½

Calories per portion (without pasta) 295

Protein 29 g

Carbohydrate 31.1 g

Fat 6 g

Oven-Baked Ham

Baked ham is a great family favorite, especially as a celebration centerpiece. This one is baked with roasted vegetables and herbs and has a lovely sticky glaze made with reduced-sugar apricot jelly. The recipe provides four normal-size portions with plenty of leftovers.

- 1 (3-pound) unsmoked ham joint
- 4 large carrots, halved lengthwise
- 1 pound baby new or waxy potatoes
- 1 pound beets, trimmed and scrubbed, halved if large
- About 6 fresh rosemary sprigs
- Low-fat nonstick cooking spray
- 2 tablespoons whole-grain mustard
- 2 tablespoons reduced-sugar apricot jelly

Preheat oven to 350°F.

Pat the ham dry with paper towels. Using the tip of a sharp knife, make deep slashes across the fat, then place in a roasting pan.

Arrange the carrots, potatoes, and beets around the ham. Tuck in the rosemary sprigs and spritz the vegetables generously with cooking spray.

Mix the mustard with the apricot jelly in a small bowl and set aside.

Bake the ham for 1 hour. Remove the pan from the oven and brush half of the mustard mixture over the ham. Return to the oven and cook for 40 minutes more, basting with the remaining mustard mixture after 20 minutes.

Transfer the ham to a carving board and cover with foil. Leave to stand in a warm place for 10 minutes before carving thinly to serve. Keep the vegetables warm for serving with the ham.

Serves 4 (with leftovers)

WLS portion ½

Calories per portion (assuming 4 ounces of ham per serving) 350

Protein 34 g

Carbohydrate 40.5 g

Fat 5.8 g

Crustless Quiche with Ham

If you're looking for a portable portion of food to take on a picnic, to the park, to the office, or simply out into the yard or garden, here is a winning recipe that travels well and is bursting with protein and other great nutrients. In the basic recipe, the ham is chopped and mixed with other savory ingredients, but you can use wafer-thin cooked ham slices to line the muffin molds or flan dish instead to give a meaty and frilly "crust" to the quiche.

- 6 large eggs, beaten
- 2 tablespoons snipped fresh chives or sliced scallions
- 4 ounces wafer-thin cooked ham slices, chopped
- ½ onion, finely chopped
- Salt and freshly ground black pepper
- Low-fat nonstick cooking spray
- 4 Babybel light cheeses, each cut into 6 pieces

Preheat oven to 350°F.

Mix the eggs with the chives, ham, onion, and salt and pepper to taste.

Spritz six holes of a deep muffin tray or medium flan or quiche dish with cooking spray. Pour in the egg mixture, ensuring that the ham and onion are equally distributed throughout. Divide the cheese pieces among the muffin cups or quiche dish, lightly pressing them into the egg mixture.

Bake for 25 to 28 minutes or until the muffin quiches or large quiche is well risen and lightly browned but still slightly wobbly in texture. (It will continue to cook after being removed from the oven. This gives a creamy rather than overcooked, rubbery texture.)

Allow to cool, then chill until ready to serve.

continued ▶

Serve the muffin-size quiches individually or cut the large quiche into wedges for serving.

Serves 6   *Protein 14.1 g*

WLS portion ½ to 1   *Carbohydrate 0.3 g*

Calories per portion 152   *Fat 10.4 g*

Sweet Potato, Broccolini, and Bacon Hash

Sweet potatoes and broccolini make a nutritious combination packed with vitamins, minerals, and fiber. This recipe would make a wonderful late-morning brunch dish over a holiday weekend like Easter, or a light main meal dish anytime.

- 1½ pounds sweet potatoes, peeled and chopped
- 8 ounces broccolini, halved lengthwise
- Low-fat nonstick cooking spray
- 6 dry-cured bacon slices, chopped
- 1 red onion, sliced
- Freshly ground black pepper
- 4 poached eggs, for serving

Bring a saucepan of water to a boil. Place the sweet potatoes in a steamer basket and steam over the boiling water for 10 minutes. Add the broccolini and steam for 4 minutes more, until both vegetables are just tender.

Meanwhile, generously spritz a pan with cooking spray. Heat over medium heat, add the bacon, onion, and pepper to taste, and cook until the onions have softened.

Add the steamed sweet potatoes and broccolini to the pan, patting them down with a wooden spoon, and cook for 10 to 15 minutes, stirring once or twice to break up the golden crust that forms on the bottom.

Spoon the hash onto four warmed serving plates and top each serving with a poached egg.

Serves 4

WLS portion ½ to 1

Calories per portion 335

Protein 22.5 g

Carbohydrate 41.8 g

Fat 9.6 g

Pasta-Free Lasagna

Vegetarian / Suitable for Freezing

Many bariatric patients find they are intolerant of pasta after surgery, which means much-loved traditional favorites like lasagna are off the menu. Until now, that is. Simply replace the pasta sheets with slices of eggplant and zucchini, and you have the makings of an authentic alternative. This recipe uses extra-lean ground beef, but if you want to make a vegetarian version, simply use a ground meat substitute (like ground Quorn) instead. Serve with a salad of seasonal vegetables alongside.

- 1 large eggplant, thinly sliced lengthwise
- 2 zucchini, thinly sliced lengthwise
- Low-fat nonstick cooking spray
- Salt and freshly ground black pepper
- 14 ounces extra-lean ground beef
- 1 onion, finely chopped
- 1 garlic clove, crushed
- 2 cups sliced mushrooms
- 1 (14-ounce) can chopped tomatoes with herbs
- 1 tablespoon tomato paste
- 2 tablespoons Worcestershire sauce
- 2 ½ tablespoons cornstarch
- Generous 2 cups low-fat milk
- 1 (4-ounce) ball light mozzarella, thinly sliced

Preheat broiler to high. Place the eggplant and zucchini slices on a nonstick baking sheet (or a baking sheet lined with a silicone mat) and generously spritz with cooking spray. Add salt and pepper to taste and broil until cooked through, about 6 minutes, turning once. Set aside while you make the filling.

Preheat oven to 400°F.

Place the beef in a large nonstick pan and cook over medium heat until browned. Add the onion, garlic, mushrooms, tomatoes, tomato paste, Worcestershire sauce, and salt and pepper to taste, mixing well. Bring to a boil, reduce the heat to maintain a simmer, and simmer for about 20 minutes until cooked and slightly thickened.

Meanwhile, in a small saucepan, combine the cornstarch with the milk and salt and pepper to taste, whisking well. Bring to a boil, whisking constantly, until smooth and thickened.

To assemble the lasagna, spoon half of the beef mixture into a large ovenproof dish. Top with half of the eggplant and zucchini slices. Top with half of the prepared sauce and half of the mozzarella slices. Repeat with the remaining meat, vegetables, sauce, and mozzarella.

Bake for about 45 minutes until golden. Allow to stand for 5 minutes before serving.

Serves 4

WLS portion ½

Calories per portion 335

Protein 37.1 g

Carbohydrate 27.3 g

Fat 8.7 g

Steak with Pepper Salsa

This summer outdoor barbecue special is also perfect for indoor broiling. This is a steak recipe that celebrates all the best of summer eating with tomatoes, red bell peppers, and oregano. The rump steak can be substituted for other steak cuts that may be more tender, like filet, if preferred, but adjust the cooking times accordingly.

- 1 red bell pepper, cored, seeded, and quartered
- 1 plum tomato
- 1 teaspoon balsamic vinegar
- 1 tablespoon chopped fresh oregano leaves
- ½ green chili, seeded and finely chopped
- Salt and freshly ground black pepper
- 2 (6-ounce) lean rump steaks
- Lettuce leaves, for serving (optional)

Preheat the broiler. Broil the bell pepper pieces skin-side up for about 10 minutes. Add the tomato after about 5 minutes, and cook until the skins of the peppers and tomato are blackened. Place both in a plastic bag for a few minutes until the skins are loosened. Peel off the skins, seed the tomato, and chop both the tomato and pepper flesh finely.

Place the tomato and pepper in a small bowl with the vinegar, oregano, chili, and salt and black pepper to taste. Mix well to combine.

Heat a griddle pan over medium-high heat until hot. Add the steaks to the pan and cook, turning occasionally, for 4 to 6 minutes for rare, 8 to 10 minutes for medium, and 10 to 12 minutes for well-done. Alternatively, grill the steaks over medium-hot coals to your level of doneness.

Serve the steaks with the salsa and some salad leaves, if desired.

Serves 2
WLS portion ½
Calories per portion 250

Protein 39.5 g
Carbohydrate 6.2 g
Fat 7.6 g

Pollock and Shrimp Biryani

When the weather turns colder, this is just the kind of warming spicy dish to turn to. This recipe is made with pollock but any other firm white fish may be substituted. It makes a great standby since many of the items come from the freezer.

- Low-fat nonstick cooking spray
- 1 onion, chopped
- 2 tablespoons Indian-style curry paste
- ½ teaspoon whole cumin seeds
- 1 (14-ounce) package frozen pollock, cut into bite-size pieces
- ⅔ cup frozen shelled shrimp

- 4 cups frozen or leftover cooked long-grain rice (see tip, below)
- 4 ounces frozen peas or baby peas
- 2 tablespoons chopped fresh cilantro leaves (optional)
- Salt and freshly ground black pepper

Generously spritz a large skillet with cooking spray. Heat over medium-high heat, add the onion, and cook gently until softened, about 3 minutes.

Stir in the curry paste and cumin seeds and cook for a few seconds.

Add the pollock and shrimp, stirring them into the mixture. Cook over medium-low heat, stirring often, for 4 to 5 minutes. Add a splash of water, if the pan is drying out.

Add the rice, peas, cilantro (if using), and salt and pepper to taste. Cook, stirring frequently, for 6 to 8 minutes, or until the rice is piping hot and the fish is cooked; the flesh will be opaque and should flake easily.

Serve immediately in warmed bowls.

Serves 4

WLS portion ½

Calories per portion 375

Protein 28.5 g

Carbohydrate 49.3 g

Fat 6.4 g

continued ▶

TIP

If you wish to use freshly cooked rice, cook 1 cup raw long-grain rice in lightly salted water for 12 minutes. Drain, then add to the fish mixture, but reduce the cooking time to 3 to 4 minutes.

Cod on a Pepper Bed

Here's a stir-fry recipe that's more likely to suit early post-ops than are the all-in-one-pan versions. The cod is lightly broiled until tender and opaque, and is therefore easily digestible. It's then served on a colorful bed of bell peppers and snow peas or sugar snap peas with carrots and bean sprouts.

- 4 (5-ounce) skinless wild Alaska Pacific cod fillets
- Finely grated zest and juice of 1 lime
- 6 scallions, thinly sliced
- Low-fat nonstick cooking spray
- 2 red bell peppers, cored, seeded, and finely sliced
- 2 yellow bell peppers, cored, seeded, and finely sliced
- 4 ounces snow peas or sugar snap peas, halved
- 1 large carrot, peeled and sliced into julienne strips
- 2 cups bean sprouts
- Soy sauce
- Freshly ground black pepper

Preheat the broiler. Cover the broiler rack with foil and arrange the cod fillets on top. Sprinkle the fish with the lime zest, lime juice, and a few slices of scallion. Broil for 6 to 8 minutes until the flesh of the fish is opaque and flakes easily.

Meanwhile, generously spritz a wok or large nonstick skillet with cooking spray and heat over medium-high heat until hot. Add the bell peppers, remaining scallions, snow peas, and carrot. Stir-fry for 3 to 4 minutes. Add the bean sprouts and stir-fry for 1 minute more.

Distribute the stir-fry among four plates and top each serving with a cod fillet. Serve, seasoned with soy sauce and black pepper to taste.

Serves 4

WLS portion ½

Calories per portion 236

Protein 31.7 g

Carbohydrate 20.5 g

Fat 3.8 g

Salmon with Chunky Ratatouille

Enjoy a taste of French cuisine by topping chunky vegetable ratatouille with a broiled fillet of salmon flavored with fresh Mediterranean herbs. This typical rustic vegetable dish is also delicious with broiled chicken.

- 4 (5-ounce) skinless wild Alaskan salmon fillets
- Finely grated zest and juice of 1 lemon
- 2 tablespoons chopped fresh herbs (such as a mix of parsley, chervil, chives, and thyme)
- Low-fat nonstick cooking spray
- 2 red onions, chopped
- 2 garlic cloves, chopped
- 1 medium eggplant, cut into chunks
- 2 zucchini, sliced crosswise
- ¼ cup tomato paste
- 12 cherry tomatoes, halved
- Generous ½ cup vegetable stock
- Salt and freshly ground black pepper

Put the salmon in a shallow glass baking dish and add the lemon zest, lemon juice, and herbs. Turn to coat, then cover and leave to marinate while making the ratatouille.

Generously spritz a saucepan with cooking spray. Heat over low heat until hot, then add the onions and garlic. Cover and cook for about 5 minutes to soften.

Add the eggplant, zucchini, tomato paste, cherry tomatoes, and stock and cook, stirring occasionally, for about 15 minutes, until the vegetables are tender. Season with salt and pepper.

Meanwhile, preheat the broiler. Arrange the salmon fillets on the broiler rack and start to broil when the ratatouille has been cooking for 6 to 7 minutes. Broil the fish for 6 to 8 minutes (depending on thickness—assume 10 minutes of cooking per inch of thickness), basting occasionally with the lemon and herb mixture.

Spoon the ratatouille onto warmed plates and top each portion with a salmon fillet to serve.

Serves 4   *Protein 35.6 g*

WLS portion ½   *Carbohydrate 18 g*

Calories per portion 320   *Fat 11.1 g*

Wild Alaskan Salmon Celebration Roast

This show-stopping salmon dish has a crust flavored with orange zest, rosemary, and dried fruit. Perfect for a special occasion, it's delicious with baby new or waxy potatoes and grilled zucchini.

- Low-fat nonstick cooking spray
- 1 (22-ounce) wild Alaska salmon fillet, in one piece
- 2/3 cup dry couscous
- 2/3 cup hot vegetable stock, heated
- Zest and juice of 1 orange, plus 1 orange, sliced
- 1/4 cup seedless raisins
- 1/4 cup chopped dried soft apricots
- 1/4 cup dried cranberries
- 1/4 cup sliced almonds
- 2 teaspoons chopped fresh rosemary leaves, plus fresh rosemary sprigs
- Salt and freshly ground black pepper

Preheat oven to 300°F.

Generously spritz a large roasting pan with cooking spray and place the salmon on top.

Put the couscous in a heatproof bowl and add the hot vegetable stock, orange zest, and orange juice. Cover and leave to soak and expand for about 10 minutes.

Add the raisins, apricots, cranberries, almonds, chopped rosemary, and salt and pepper to taste, mixing well. Spoon the mixture over the salmon, then cover the roasting pan with a sheet of foil.

Bake in the center of the oven for 20 minutes, then remove the foil and arrange the orange slices and rosemary sprigs on top. Return the pan to the oven and cook, uncovered, for 10 to 15 minutes more, or until the fish flakes easily.

Serve hot.

Serves 4

WLS portion 1/3 to 1/2

Calories per portion 454

Protein 37.8 g

Carbohydrate 41.5 g

Fat 15.5 g

Thai Steamed Salmon

In this dish, salmon fillets are marinated with cilantro, ginger, mint, lime juice, and chilies and then steamed for a typical Thai taste. Serve with brown basmati rice or rice noodles and perhaps a small side serving of steamed green beans or bok choy.

- 1 bunch fresh cilantro
- 12 fresh mint leaves
- ½ teaspoon salt
- 1 garlic cloves, crushed
- 2 green chilies, seeded and chopped
- 3 tablespoons fresh lime juice
- 1 tablespoon Splenda granulated sweetener
- 1 teaspoon chopped peeled fresh ginger
- 1 tablespoon nam pla fish sauce
- 4 (4-ounce) skinless and boneless salmon fillets

In a food processor, combine the cilantro, mint, salt, garlic, and chilies and process to make a rough paste. Add the lime juice, sweetener, ginger, and fish sauce and process until fairly smooth. Spoon the paste into a heatproof bowl and add the salmon. Cover and leave to marinate for at least 20 minutes.

Boil some water in the base of a steamer. Place the bowl with the marinated salmon on top and steam for 6 to 8 minutes, or until the fish is cooked through and flakes easily.

Serve immediately.

Serves 4
WLS portion ½
Calories per portion 240

Protein 25.7 g
Carbohydrate 2 g
Fat 13.6 g

Tuna Steaks with Mango-Avocado Salad

An accompaniment of rich avocado with juicy mango and herbs makes this simple dish a special treat, and it can be ready and on the table in under 20 minutes.

For the salad

- 2 ripe mangoes, pitted, peeled, and chopped
- 1 large ripe avocado, pitted, peeled, and chopped
- ½ red chili, seeded and finely chopped
- 3 tablespoons chopped fresh mint leaves
- 2 tablespoons chopped fresh basil leaves
- 2 tablespoons chopped fresh cilantro leaves
- Zest of 1 lime
- Juice of 2 limes
- Salt and freshly ground white pepper

For the tuna

- 4 (4-ounce) fresh tuna steaks, about 1 inch thick
- Low-fat nonstick cooking spray
- Salt and freshly ground white pepper
- Lime wedges, for serving

To prepare the salad: Place the mango, avocado, chili, herbs, lime zest, and lime juice in a bowl with salt and white pepper to taste. Mix together and set aside.

To prepare the tuna: Place a skillet or griddle pan over high heat. Generously spritz the tuna steaks with cooking spray and season with salt and white pepper. Place the steaks in the skillet and cook for 1 to 1½ minutes on each side for rare, or 2 minutes per side for medium.

Serve the tuna with the mango-avocado salad and lime wedges alongside.

Serves 4

WLS portion ½

Calorie per portion 353

Protein 59 g

Carbohydrate 8.9 g

Fat 8.5 g

Warm Leek, Smoked Trout, and Potato Salad

Here's a beautifully elegant appetizer size salad that is also good as a buffet table addition. If you wish to serve as an entrée (or for large appetites), double the quantities. Choose small to medium leeks that have a tender texture and long white necks, and use reduced-fat crème fraîche to keep the fat content low.

- 4 small to medium leeks, white parts only, well washed and halved into equal lengths (8 total pieces)
- 3 ounces peeled waxy potatoes, cubed
- ¼ cup reduced-fat crème fraîche
- 2 teaspoons creamed horseradish
- 4 scallions, finely sliced
- 1 small bunch fresh chives, finely snipped
- Zest and juice of 1 lemon
- Salt and freshly ground black pepper
- 2 smoked trout fillets, skinned and flaked
- Arugula or watercress leaves, for garnish

Bring a saucepan of water to a boil. Cook the leeks for 8 minutes, then drain and set aside, but keep warm.

Meanwhile, place the potatoes in a saucepan with enough water to cover and bring to a boil. Cook until tender, about 10 minutes. Drain and set aside, but keep warm.

In a small bowl, combine the crème fraîche, horseradish, scallions, chives, lemon zest, lemon juice, and salt and pepper to taste. Mix well.

To serve, place 2 leeks on each serving plate, add a small spoonful of the warm potatoes and some of the flaked smoked trout, and drizzle with the crème fraîche dressing. Garnish with a few arugula or watercress leaves and serve while still warm.

Serves 4

WLS portion ½ to ¾

Calories per portion 125

Protein 10.4 g

Carbohydrate 11.3 g

Fat 4.4 g

Salade Niçoise

This salad, made with tuna, eggs, green beans, and peas, is endlessly versatile. It makes a wonderful light summer lunch for friends and yet can be packed for a desktop lunch or picnic.

- 8 ounces new or small waxy potatoes, halved
- 4 large eggs
- 8 ounces green beans, trimmed
- 4 ounces fresh shelled or frozen peas
- 1 (7.5-ounce) can tuna in water, drained and flaked

- 12 ripe olives
- 4 anchovy fillets, halved
- 1 small shallot, very finely chopped
- 5 tablespoons fat-free French dressing
- Salt and freshly ground black pepper

Place the potatoes in a saucepan and add enough water to cover. Bring to a boil and cook the potatoes until tender, about 15 minutes. Drain and set aside.

Meanwhile, bring a small saucepan of water to a boil. Add the eggs and cook until just hard-boiled but not dry, about 7 minutes. Rinse under running water for 5 minutes until cool, then remove the eggshells and halve the eggs. Set aside.

In the meantime, bring a large saucepan of salted water to a boil. Blanch the green beans and peas for 2 minutes. Drain, then shock under cold water and drain again.

In a large bowl, mix the potatoes with the eggs, green beans, peas, tuna, olives, and anchovies.

Mix the shallot with the French dressing and salt and pepper to taste. Pour the dressing over the salad mixture and toss gently to coat. Serve immediately.

Serves 4   *Protein 19.7 g*
WLS portion ½   *Carbohydrate 16.5 g*
Calories per portion 220   *Fat 8.1 g*

Italian Bean and Sardine Salad

This colorful red, white, and green salad mixture has a summery flavor courtesy of the basil. It can be made with any fat-free or low-fat dressing, but the tomato and pepper dressing (see the tip at the end of the recipe) is especially good. To save time, use canned or bottled red bell peppers, packed in brine or water rather than oil to avoid excess fat.

- ¾ cup cooked or canned cannellini beans, drained and rinsed if canned
- ½ cup chopped roasted red bell pepper
- 1 cup shredded or torn romaine lettuce
- 1 (4.5-ounce) can skinless and boneless sardines
- 2 tablespoons fat-free or low-fat Italian dressing, or 2 tablespoons tomato and pepper dressing (see tip, below)
- 1 teaspoon finely chopped fresh basil leaves, or ½ teaspoon dried basil or oregano
- Salt and freshly ground black pepper

Place the beans in a bowl with the bell pepper and lettuce and toss to mix. Spoon onto a serving plate and top with the sardines.

Mix the dressing with the basil and salt and black pepper to taste. Spoon the dressing over the sardines and bean salad to serve.

Serves 1

WLS portion ½

Calories per portion 260

Protein 34.8 g

Carbohydrate 15.1 g

Fat 5.1 g

TIP

This bean salad is especially good when tossed with tomato and pepper dressing: Mix one 6-ounce can tomato paste with 1 very finely chopped roasted bell pepper, 2 tablespoons red wine vinegar, 2 tablespoons water, 1 crushed garlic clove, 1 teaspoon chopped fresh basil or ½ teaspoon dried basil, and salt and pepper to taste. Chill in the refrigerator until ready to use. The dressing will keep in an airtight container for up to 1 week.

Greek Salad

Vegetarian

This has to be one of the most popular salads with its mix of lettuce, cucumber, olives, tomatoes, feta, and herbs. You can add a few anchovies to the mix, if desired. A little crusty bread would be perfect to mop up the juices, if you can tolerate it.

- 1 head romaine lettuce, shredded
- ½ cucumber, peeled and diced
- 1 red onion, thinly sliced
- 4 tomatoes, coarsely chopped or sliced
- 8 ounces low-fat feta cheese, cut into cubes
- 4 anchovy fillets, halved (optional)
- 12 ripe olives, pitted
- 4 tablespoons fat-free dressing of choice
- 2 teaspoons fresh thyme leaves

Layer the lettuce, cucumber, onion, tomatoes, feta, anchovies (if using), and olives in four thick glass tumblers or serving dishes.

Spoon 1 tablespoon of the fat-free dressing over each portion and sprinkle with some of the fresh thyme leaves. Serve lightly chilled.

Serves 4

WLS portion ½

Calories per portion 180

Protein 13.7 g

Carbohydrate 10.4 g

Fat 9.3 g

Warm Green Bean, Halloumi, and Potato Salad

Vegetarian

This is a filling, substantial salad, ideal for a main meal. It is made with halloumi cheese, a firm, slightly springy white cheese from Cyprus, made with sheep's and goat's milk (although now sometimes with cow's milk). Halloumi has a texture similar to mozzarella but a stronger, saltier flavor. When cooked, it keeps its firm texture due to its high melting point. Mixed with herbs and olives in this salad, it adds a welcome taste of the Mediterranean.

- 8 ounces small new or waxy potatoes, sliced
- 8 ounces haricots verts, trimmed
- ⅓ cup fat-free French dressing
- 2 ounces baby capers, rinsed
- 2 tablespoons chopped fresh mint leaves
- 1 tablespoon chopped fresh dill
- 12 ripe olives, pitted
- 5 ounces cherry tomatoes, halved
- Salt and freshly ground black pepper
- Low-fat nonstick cooking spray
- 8 ounces reduced-fat or light halloumi cheese

Place the potatoes in a medium saucepan and add water to cover. Bring to a boil and cook the potatoes until tender, 12 to 15 minutes. Drain and set aside.

Meanwhile, bring a saucepan of water to a boil. Add the haricots verts and cook for 2 minutes. Drain and set aside.

In a large bowl, mix the French dressing with the capers, mint, dill, and olives. Add the potatoes, haricots verts, tomatoes, and salt and pepper to taste, mixing well.

continued ▶

Generously spritz a nonstick skillet or griddle pan with low-fat spray and heat until hot. Add the halloumi cheese and cook for 1 minute on each side until golden brown. Remove and cut into bite-size cubes. Add the cheese cubes to the salad and mix gently to serve.

Serves 4

WLS portion ½

Calories per portion 215

Protein 14.9 g

Carbohydrate 14.3 g

Fat 10.4 g

Warm Goat Cheese with Pear and Pecan Salad

Vegetarian

Here's a warming dish bursting with the fresh flavors of autumn or the festive Christmas season. Sliced pears, pecans, haricots verts, and baby greens are tossed with a cranberry-chili dressing and topped with cooked goat cheese. Bariatrics who have poor tolerance of sugars might like to use a no-sugar-added cranberry sauce (see page 165).

- 4 ounces haricots verts, trimmed
- 4 ounces semifirm goat cheese
- 2 ripe pears
- 2 tablespoons lemon juice
- 2 tablespoons cranberry sauce
- Pinch of ground cinnamon
- 1 tablespoon low-fat spread or light butter
- Salt and freshly ground black pepper
- 7 ounces mixed baby salad leaves
- 1 small red chili, seeded and very thinly sliced
- ¼ cup pecans

Bring a saucepan of water to a boil. Add the haricots verts and cook for 2 minutes. Drain and shock under cold water, then drain again.

Meanwhile, cut the goat cheese into chunks. Quarter the pears, remove the core, then slice each quarter into thin slices.

Place the lemon juice, cranberry sauce, cinnamon, and low-fat spread in a heavy-bottomed skillet. Add the pear slices and salt and pepper to taste and cook for 2 to 3 minutes until the pears are beginning to soften.

Toss the cheese into the pan and cook for 2 to 3 minutes more, until the cheese begins to soften.

continued ▶

Meanwhile, toss the salad leaves with the haricots verts, chili, and pecans and divide among four plates. Top each with an equal quantity of the hot pear-and-cheese mixture. Serve immediately.

Serves 4　　　　　　　　*Protein 5.9 g*
WLS portion ½　　　　*Carbohydrate 13.7 g*
Calories per portion 180　*Fat 11.5 g*

Chickpea and Broccoli Frittata

Vegetarian

This popular Italian-style omelet is a tasty and nutritious way of getting protein into your diet post-op. This one is given an extra protein boost with chickpeas, but you could substitute cooked chicken, ham, or flaked fish for a quick lunch or brunch dish. Serve with a light side salad, if desired. Use the remaining chickpeas to make a small batch of hummus (see page 66).

- 6 ounces broccoli, trimmed
- Low-fat nonstick cooking spray
- ½ red onion, finely chopped
- 1 small red bell pepper, cored, seeded, and chopped
- 1 garlic clove, crushed
- ½ teaspoon smoked paprika
- ½ (14-ounce) can chickpeas, drained and rinsed
- 2 tablespoons chopped fresh cilantro leaves
- 7 large eggs
- Salt and freshly ground black pepper

Preheat oven to 375°F.

Bring a saucepan of water to a boil. Add the broccoli and cook for 2 to 3 minutes or until almost tender. Drain, chop coarsely, and set aside.

Generously spritz a large skillet with cooking spray. Heat over moderate heat, then add the onion and bell pepper and cook for 5 minutes until soft.

Add the garlic, paprika, and chickpeas and cook for 2 minutes more. Add the cilantro, mixing well.

Generously spritz a ceramic baking dish, about 10 x 5 inches, or a 7-inch springform pan, with cooking spray. Spread the chickpea mixture over the base of the prepared dish. Top with the chopped broccoli.

continued ▶

Beat the eggs with salt and pepper to taste and pour over the broccoli.

Bake for about 25 minutes or until golden and set.

Serve warm or cold, cut into wedges.

Serves 4	*Protein 18.6 g*
WLS portion ½	*Carbohydrate 8.8 g*
Calories per portion 230	*Fat 13.5 g*

Pumpkin, Bean, and Tomato Risotto

Vegetarian

Here's a lovely risotto dish made extra easy by the addition of baked beans. The final sprinkling of Parmesan and torn fresh basil give the dish an authentic Italian flavor.

- 2 tablespoons low-fat spread or light butter
- 1 onion, finely chopped
- 11 ounces pumpkin, peeled, seeded, and cut into bite-size pieces
- 2 garlic cloves, crushed
- Salt and freshly ground black pepper
- 1¼ cups raw arborio rice
- Generous 3½ cups vegetable stock, heated
- 1 (14-ounce) can reduced-sugar and low-sodium baked beans in tomato sauce
- 3 tomatoes, peeled and chopped
- 3 tablespoons torn fresh basil
- 3 tablespoons grated Parmesan

Melt the low-fat spread in a large nonstick skillet over medium-high heat. Add the onion and cook for 3 to 4 minutes or until soft.

Stir in the pumpkin, garlic, and salt and pepper to taste and cook for 8 to 10 minutes or until the pumpkin is slightly softened.

Add the rice and stir until it is coated in the juices. Stir in about ½ cup of the hot stock and cook until it has been absorbed by the rice.

Add another ladleful of the stock to the rice and cook over medium heat, stirring constantly, until the liquid has been absorbed. Add another ladleful of the stock and continue cooking and stirring, repeating the additions for 15 to 18 minutes, or until the rice is tender. You may not need all of the stock.

continued ▶

Stir in the beans and tomatoes, bring to a boil, and add 2 tablespoons of the basil, mixing well.

Serve the risotto in bowls, sprinkled with the Parmesan and the remaining torn basil.

Serves 4

WLS portion ½

Calories per portion 458

Protein 15.4 g

Carbohydrate 84.9 g

Fat 6.1 g

Israeli Couscous with Roasted Vegetables

Vegan / Vegetarian

You could use ordinary couscous for this dish, but Israeli couscous has a much nuttier flavor and more satisfying texture. The whole-wheat variety also works well here. The vegetables could be mixed with cooked chicken, cheese, or chickpeas for additional protein, if desired. This is a versatile dish that can be eaten hot or cold.

- 1 medium eggplant
- 2 medium zucchini
- 1 green bell pepper, cored and seeded
- 1 yellow bell pepper, cored and seeded
- 1 large sweet potato, peeled
- 2 red onions, cut into wedges
- 1 to 2 teaspoons harissa paste
- Salt and freshly ground black pepper
- Low-fat nonstick cooking spray
- 1 pound cherry tomatoes
- Sprigs of fresh thyme
- 10 ounces whole-wheat Israeli couscous
- Vegetable stock

Preheat oven to 450°F.

Cut the eggplant, zucchini, bell peppers, and sweet potato into bite-size pieces and mix with the onions, harissa paste, and salt and black pepper to taste. Transfer to a large nonstick baking pan and spritz generously with cooking spray. Roast for 30 minutes.

Remove from the oven and add the tomatoes and thyme. Turn the vegetables over with a spatula and spritz again with a little more cooking spray. Return to the oven and cook for 10 to 15 minutes more, or until the vegetables are tender.

continued ▶

Meanwhile, cook the couscous according to the package instructions, using vegetable stock in place of water as called for.

Serve the roasted vegetables, warm or cold, over the cooked couscous.

Serves 6

WLS portion ½

Calories per portion 260

Protein 10 g

Carbohydrate 51.6 g

Fat 2.3 g

Nutty Amaretti-Stuffed Peaches

Vegetarian

Nothing sings out summer more than juicy peaches, and white-fleshed ones are particularly succulent and sweet. This delicious and quick recipe makes the most of them with a filling of creamy cheese mixed with crushed amaretti cookies. When fresh peaches aren't in season, replace them with canned peach halves in natural juice (not sugar syrup).

- 4 fresh ripe peaches, skinned, if desired
- ¾ ounce (about 10) small amaretti cookies
- 7 ounces low-fat cream cheese or other soft cheese
- 2 tablespoons Splenda granulated sweetener
- 1 tablespoon sliced almonds, toasted
- 2 teaspoons low-sugar fruit nectar (such as Goya mango nectar)
- Mint leaves, for garnish (optional)

Halve the peaches and remove and discard the pits.

Crush the amaretti and place in a bowl with the cream cheese, sweetener, almonds, and nectar. Mix well to combine.

Carefully spoon some of the amaretti mixture into the center of each peach half.

Serve garnished with mint leaves, if desired.

Serves 4

WLS portion ½

Calories per portion 120

Protein 8.4 g

Carbohydrate 15.8 g

Fat 2.8 g

Apple and Pineapple Kebabs with Ginger-Yogurt Dip
Vegetarian

These juicy fruit kebabs with a zingy dip make the perfect end to any meal. Pink Lady apples are a good choice since they are perfectly pink, crunchy, and sweet. If you have trouble digesting pineapple, omit it and double the quantity of apples.

- 1 Pink Lady apple, cored and cut into 12 wedges
- ¼ small pineapple, peeled, cored, and cut into cubes
- 4 tablespoons sugar-free or reduced sugar apricot jelly
- ⅔ cup fat-free Greek yogurt
- 2 teaspoons finely grated peeled fresh ginger
- A few fresh mint leaves, roughly torn

Thread the apple and pineapple pieces onto four skewers, alternating the fruit. Brush with 1 tablespoon of the jelly.

Heat a griddle pan until very hot, add the skewers and cook, turning frequently, for 4 to 5 minutes, until charbroiled. Remove and allow to cool slightly.

Meanwhile, in a small bowl, combine the yogurt with the remaining 3 tablespoons of jelly and the ginger, mixing well.

Serve the kebabs while still warm (but do not serve too soon, as the fruit will be very hot), topped with a few torn mint leaves and with the yogurt dip alongside.

Serves 2

WLS portion ½

Calories per portion 137

Protein 7.4 g

Carbohydrate 26.5 g

Fat 0.2 g

Apple Berry Crumble

Vegan / Vegetarian / Suitable for Freezing

A real comfort-food favorite, this dessert has been adapted so it's no longer heavy on sugar or rich in butter, but tastes just as sublime. The secret to making it bariatric-friendly is to make it loaded with fruit and light on topping. Serve plain or with low-fat and low-sugar pudding, fat-free yogurt, or light ice cream.

For the filling

- 1½ pounds cooking apples (such as Northern Spy or Pink Lady), peeled, cored, and sliced
- 1¼ cups blackberries
- 2 tablespoons Splenda granulated sweetener

For the crumble

- 1 cup all-purpose flour
- 1 cup whole-wheat flour
- 3 ounces low-fat spread or light butter
- 3 tablespoons Splenda granulated sweetener
- ¼ cup sliced almonds

Preheat oven to 400°F.

To prepare the filling: Mix the apples and blackberries with the sweetener and place in a baking dish.

To prepare the crumble: Combine the flours in a large bowl. Rub the low-fat spread into the flour until the mixture has the texture of fine bread crumbs. Stir in the sweetener and almonds. Sprinkle the crumble mixture evenly on top of the fruit.

Bake for 25 to 30 minutes or until the fruit is soft and the crumble is golden and crunchy.

Serve hot.

Serves 6

WLS portion ½

Calories per portion 232

Protein 6.3 g

Carbohydrate 34.2 g

Fat 7.8 g

Pear-Ginger Cake

Vegetarian / Suitable for Freezing

This beautifully moist cake, packed with pears and spiced with ginger, is not only wonderful plain but also served warm with low-fat pudding, fat-free Greek yogurt, or a bariatric-friendly ice cream. It's a versatile recipe that can also be made with apples and cinnamon. Try both and choose your favorite.

- Low-fat nonstick cooking spray
- 1 cup all-purpose flour
- 1 heaping tablespoon granulated Splenda sweetener
- 2 teaspoons ground ginger
- 2 teaspoons baking powder

- 3 large eggs, beaten
- 3 tablespoons low-fat milk
- 6 tablespoons low-fat spread or light butter, melted
- 2 pounds assorted pears, peeled, cored, and cut into thin slices

---

Preheat oven to 400°F.

Generously spritz a 9-inch nonstick springform pan with cooking spray.

In a large bowl, combine the flour, sweetener, ginger, and baking powder. Make a well in the center and add the eggs and milk. Whisk well, then whisk in the melted spread to combine.

Gently fold the pear slices into the batter. Spoon the batter into the prepared pan.

Bake for 30 to 35 minutes, until well-risen, firm, and golden.

Allow to cool slightly before slicing. Serve warm, or allow to cool to serve cold.

Serves 8

WLS portion ½

Calories per portion 162

Protein 4 g

Carbohydrates 30 g

Fat 4 g

VARIATION
Apple-Cinnamon Cake

Prepare the cake as above, but use a mixture of baking and dessert apples instead of the pears, and ground cinnamon instead of the ground ginger.

Banana-Walnut Tea Bread

Vegetarian / Suitable for Freezing

Many bariatric patients believe they can never enjoy a sweet treat again. I hope this recipe dispels that myth. It works on so many levels: It keeps well, provides some much-needed protein, and is low in calories, fat, and sugar. If you wish to boost the protein further, add a scoop of whey protein powder to the dry ingredients. The powder can be unflavored or flavored; if you're considering the latter, vanilla or banana flavor works very well.

- Low-fat nonstick cooking spray
- 2 ripe large bananas, mashed
- 2 large eggs, beaten
- 1½ teaspoons vanilla extract
- ½ cup plus 1 tablespoon Splenda granulated sweetener
- Generous 1 cup all-purpose flour
- Generous 1 cup ground almonds or almond flour
- 3¾ teaspoons baking powder
- Pinch of salt
- 3 tablespoons butter, melted
- ¾ cup chopped walnuts

Preheat oven to 350°F.

Spritz an 8½ × 4½ × 2½–inch nonstick loaf pan with cooking spray.

In a large bowl, mix the bananas with the eggs, vanilla, and sweetener until well combined.

In a separate bowl, mix the flour with the almonds, baking powder, and salt. Fold the dry ingredients into the banana mixture. Stir in the melted butter and the walnuts.

Spoon the batter into the prepared loaf pan and bake for 40 to 50 minutes or until a skewer inserted into the center comes out clean and not sticky.

Allow to cool on a wire rack. Cut into 16 slices and serve.

Makes 16 slices

WLS portion ½ to 1 slice

Calories per portion: 140

Protein 4 g

Carbohydrate 10.8 g

Fat 9.6 g

Pumpkin Bread

Vegetarian / Suitable for Freezing

During the fall, pumpkin bread is a must, but not the high-sugar version from pre-surgery days. This one is moist, spicy, and sweet—and most important, bariatric-friendly. It can be topped with the frosting used on the Celebratory Carrot Cake (see page 211), if desired (this will affect the nutritional value).

- Low-fat nonstick cooking spray
- 1¾ cups all-purpose flour
- 1 teaspoon baking soda
- ½ teaspoon baking powder
- 1 teaspoon ground cinnamon
- ½ teaspoon ground ginger
- ¼ teaspoon freshly grated nutmeg
- ½ teaspoon salt
- 4 tablespoons light butter
- ¾ cup Splenda granulated sweetener
- ¼ cup olive oil
- 1 cup pureed pumpkin, or ½ (15-ounce) can pure pumpkin
- 2 large eggs
- ¼ cup water
- ⅓ cup raisins

Preheat oven to 350°F.

Generously spritz an 8½ × 4½ × 2½–inch nonstick loaf pan with cooking spray.

In a large bowl, mix the flour with the baking soda, baking powder, cinnamon, ginger, nutmeg, and salt.

Using a hand mixer, whisk the butter in a bowl with the sweetener and oil until light and fluffy, about 2 minutes.

Blend the pumpkin into the butter mixture, and then add the eggs, one at a time, and whisk until well combined. Slowly add the flour mixture and the water and mix well, then fold in the raisins. Spoon into the prepared loaf pan.

continued ▶

Bake for 60 to 75 minutes or until a skewer inserted into the center comes out clean and not sticky.

Allow to stand for 10 minutes in the pan, then turn out the loaf onto a wire rack to cool completely. Cut into 16 slices and serve.

Makes 16 slices

WLS portion ½ to 1 slice

Calories per portion 104

Protein 2.5 g

Carbohydrate 12.6 g

Fat 5 g

TIP

Vary this cake mixture by adding ½ cup chopped pecans, walnuts, dried cranberries, or sugar-free chocolate chips to this recipe instead of the raisins. Fold into the prepared cake mixture just before baking.

Cream Cheese–Frosted Cupcakes

Vegetarian

That old favorite cupcake with cream cheese frosting has been given a makeover to make it bariatric-friendly. This one scores on all levels: it's low in fat and sugar and has a good quantity of protein for a special treat.

For the cupcakes

- 1½ cups all-purpose flour
- 2½ teaspoons baking powder
- ½ cup plus 2 tablespoons Splenda granulated sweetener
- ¼ cup low-fat milk powder
- 3 tablespoons ground rice
- 2 large eggs, beaten
- Generous ½ cup vegetable oil
- ¼ cup low-fat milk
- ½ cup water, plus more as needed
- 1 teaspoon vanilla extract
- Dash of salt

For the frosting

- ⅔ cup low-fat cream cheese or soft cheese
- 4 teaspoons Splenda granulated sweetener
- ¼ teaspoon vanilla extract
- Sugar-free chocolate cutouts or fresh berries, for garnish

To make the cupcakes: Preheat oven to 350°F.

Sift the flour and baking powder into a bowl. Stir in the sweetener, milk powder, and ground rice.

In a separate bowl, mix the eggs, oil, milk, water, vanilla, and salt. Stir the egg mixture into the dry ingredients with a wooden spoon. The mixture should have a soft dropping consistency. If not, add another 1 tablespoon water. Divide equally among 14 paper-lined muffin tin cups or silicone cupcake molds set on a baking sheet.

continued ▶

Bake for 15 to 20 minutes until well risen and light golden. Allow to cool on a wire rack.

To make the frosting: In a bowl, beat the cream cheese with the sweetener and vanilla until light and fluffy. Transfer to a piping bag or a zip-top bag with one corner snipped.

Pipe or swirl the frosting onto the tops of the cooled cakes, then decorate with sugar-free chocolate cutouts or fresh berries.

The cupcakes will keep in an airtight container in the refrigerator for up to 2 days.

Makes 14 cupcakes

WLS portion ½ to 1 cupcake

Calories per portion 143

Protein 4.8 g

Carbohydrate 13.1 g

Fat 7.8 g

Celebratory Carrot Cake

Vegetarian

Birthdays and other celebrations don't go away just because you've had weight-loss surgery, so there are still temptations with the cakes and other treats offered on these occasions. Indeed, you might want to mark your own surgery anniversary (or "surgi-versary") with something edible. It's hard, if not impossible, to find a bariatric-friendly cake for such events, so here's one that you can make and enjoy. Don't be put off by the long list of ingredients—the result is well worth the effort!

For the cake

- Low-fat nonstick cooking spray
- 1 (15-ounce) can pineapple pieces in fruit juice (not syrup)
- 2½ cups all-purpose flour
- 1 ounce vanilla- or pineapple-flavored protein powder
- 2 teaspoons baking powder
- ½ teaspoon salt
- 2 teaspoons ground cinnamon
- 3 large eggs, beaten
- 2 ounces Splenda granulated sweetener
- 4 ounces fat-free Greek yogurt
- ¼ cup water
- ¼ cup olive oil
- 2 ounces canned white beans (such as butter or cannellini), pureed
- 1 teaspoon vanilla extract
- 7 ounces grated carrot
- ½ cup shredded unsweetened coconut
- ¾ cup chopped walnuts

For the frosting

- 1½ cups fat-free cream cheese or other soft cheese
- 3 tablespoons Splenda granulated sweetener
- 3 tablespoons confectioners' sugar
- 1½ teaspoons vanilla extract
- 2 tablespoons shredded coconut, toasted
- Walnut halves, for garnish (optional)

continued ▶

To prepare the cake: Preheat oven to 350°F.

Generously spritz an 8-inch nonstick round cake pan with cooking spray. Line the base with a disc of waxed paper.

Drain the pineapple in a fine-mesh sieve set over a bowl, pressing down very well to extract as much juice as possible from the solids. Chop the pineapple solids into fine pieces. Reserve the juice in the bowl.

In a bowl, mix the flour with the protein powder, baking powder, salt, and cinnamon.

In a separate large bowl, beat the eggs with the sweetener, yogurt, water, oil, bean puree, vanilla, and ¼ cup of the reserved pineapple juice. Stir in the carrot, coconut, and drained chopped pineapple, mixing well.

Fold the flour mixture into the egg mixture until well combined. Fold in the chopped walnuts.

Spoon the batter into the prepared pan and spread evenly. Bake for 1 hour or until the top of the cake springs back when lightly pressed with a fingertip and a skewer inserted into the center comes out clean and not sticky. Allow to cool completely on a wire rack before frosting.

Meanwhile, to prepare the frosting: Beat the cream cheese with the sweetener, confectioners' sugar, and vanilla. Transfer the frosting to a piping bag or a ziptop bag with one corner snipped.

Swirl the frosting on top of the cake. Sprinkle with the toasted coconut and decorate with walnut halves, if desired.

Serves 16	*Protein 9.4 g*
WLS portion ½ to 1	*Carbohydrate 21.7 g*
Calories per portion 217	*Fat 10.9 g*

INDEX

39821657R00136

Made in the USA
Lexington, KY
12 March 2015